S0-AID-359

Teen Health Series

Eating Disorders Information For Teens, Fourth Edition

Teen Health Series

Eating Disorders Information For Teens, Fourth Edition

Health Tips About Anorexia, Bulimia,
Binge Eating, And Body Image Disorders

Including Information About Risk Factors, Prevention,
Diagnosis, Treatment, Health Consequences,
And Other Related Issues

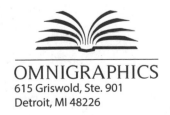

OMNIGRAPHICS
615 Griswold, Ste. 901
Detroit, MI 48226

Bibliographic Note
Because this page cannot legibly accommodate all the copyright notices, the Bibliographic Note portion of the Preface constitutes an extension of the copyright notice.

* * *

Omnigraphics
a part of Relevant Information
Keith Jones, *Managing Editor*

* * *

Copyright © 2017 Omnigraphics
ISBN 978-0-7808-1559-9
E-ISBN 978-0-7808-1560-5

Library of Congress Cataloging-in-Publication Data

Names: Omnigraphics, Inc., issuing body.

Title: Eating disorders information for teens: health tips about anorexia, bulimia, binge eating, and body image disorders including information about risk factors, prevention, diagnosis, treatment, health consequences, and other related issues.

Description: Fourth edition. | Detroit, MI: Omnigraphics, [2017] | Series: Teen health series | Audience: Grade 9 to 12. | Includes bibliographical references and index.

Identifiers: LCCN 2017010041 (print) | LCCN 2017010319 (ebook) | ISBN 9780780815599 (hardcover: alk. paper) | ISBN 9780780815605 (ebook) | ISBN 9780780815605 (eBook)

Subjects: LCSH: Eating disorders--Juvenile literature. | Eating disorders in adolescence--Juvenile literature.

Classification: LCC RC552.E18 E2836 2017 (print) | LCC RC552.E18 (ebook) | DDC 616.85/2600835--dc23

LC record available at https://lccn.loc.gov/2017010041

Electronic or mechanical reproduction, including photography, recording, or any other information storage and retrieval system for the purpose of resale is strictly prohibited without permission in writing from the publisher.

The information in this publication was compiled from the sources cited and from other sources considered reliable. While every possible effort has been made to ensure reliability, the publisher will not assume liability for damages caused by inaccuracies in the data, and makes no warranty, express or implied, on the accuracy of the information contained herein.

This book is printed on acid-free paper meeting the ANSI Z39.48 Standard. The infinity symbol that appears above indicates that the paper in this book meets that standard.

Printed in the United States

Table Of Contents

Preface

Part One: Eating Disorders And Their Risk Factors

Part Two: Understanding Eating Disorders And Body Image Disorders

DEC 2 3 2017

Part Three: Medical Consequences And Co-Occurring Concerns

Part Four: Diagnosing And Treating Eating Disorders

Part Five: Maintaining Healthy Eating And Fitness Habits

Part Six: If You Need More Information

Preface

About This Book

For many people, watching what they eat and exercising are important components of healthy lifestyles. For others, however, these concerns become extreme. Some people develop serious disruptions in eating patterns, become fixated on food worries, and experience severe distress about body weight and shape. These obsessions are characteristic of eating disorders.

Eating disorders involve extreme emotions, attitudes, and behaviors involving weight and food. The most common eating disorders include anorexia nervosa, bulimia nervosa, and other disorders. Researchers have found that eating disorders are caused by a complex interaction of genetic, biological, behavioral, psychological, and social factors. Eating disorders are common and can start at any age, but they usually start during the teen years. Females are more likely to get eating disorders than males, but statistics on the prevalence of eating disorders in the United States can vary widely. Many sufferers do not come forward for diagnosis due to embarrassment, denial, or confusion as to what their symptoms are, and eating disorders can differ vastly in the expression of symptoms and behaviors.

Eating Disorders Information For Teens, Fourth Edition, discusses the differences between healthy eating patterns and anorexia nervosa, bulimia nervosa, binge eating syndrome, emotional eating, night eating syndrome, orthorexia, pica, and other eating disorders. It explains how to recognize eating disorders, how they are diagnosed, the types of treatment available, and guidelines for relapse prevention. Facts about medical consequences, co-occurring conditions, and other diseases that may be complicated by an eating disorder are also included. A special section reports on healthy weight management and exercise plans. The book concludes with directories of resources for additional information about eating disorders, nutrition, and fitness.

How To Use This Book

This book is divided into parts and chapters. Parts focus on broad areas of interest; chapters are devoted to single topics within a part.

Part One: Eating Disorders And Their Risk Factors provides basic facts about eating disorders. It discusses how to identify healthy eating patterns, and the types of influences that can lead to disruptions in normal eating patterns. Other factors that could contribute to eating disorders such as genetics, and negative body image are also discussed. The part concludes with a chapter on weight loss and myths related to nutrition.

Part Two: Understanding Eating And Body Image Disorders provides facts about the three most common types of eating disorders: anorexia nervosa, bulimia nervosa, and binge eating disorder. It also offers information about sleep eating syndrome, pica, and other lesser-known types of eating disorders, and it discusses other related concerns, including rumination disorder, compulsive exercise and body dysmorphic disorder.

Part Three: Medical Consequences And Co-Occurring Concerns summarizes some of the most commonly experienced physical and mental problems associated with eating disorders, including the effects of inadequate nutrition, risks associated with obesity, oral health implications, osteoporosis, and fertility and pregnancy issues. It also discusses other conditions that can impact the progression and outcomes of eating disorders. The part concludes with a discussion of the impact eating disorders can have on mental health, and the potential implications associated with that.

Part Four: Diagnosing And Treating Eating Disorders talks about the common symptoms of eating disorders and how to identify someone who may be struggling with an eating disorder. Information about diagnosis and types of treatment along with medications, improving self-esteem and ways to deal with body image issues are also included.

Part Five: Maintaining Healthy Eating And Fitness Habits provides information on how to build a healthy eating style and improve your eating habits. It offers tips on how to achieve a healthy weight through good dietary habits and calorie management. The importance of good physical and mental health is also discussed. The part concludes with information on how to avoid potential relapse.

Part Six: If You Need More Information offers directories of resources for more information about eating disorders, nutrition, weight management, and physical and mental fitness.

Bibliographic Note

This volume contains documents and excerpts from publications issued by the following government agencies: Centers for Disease Control and Prevention (CDC); *Eunice Kennedy Shriver* National Institute of Child Health and Human Development (NICHD); Federal Occupational Health (FOH); Genetic and Rare Diseases Information Center (GARD); Genetics Home Reference (GHR); National Heart Lung and Blood Institute (NHLBI);

National Institute of Arthritis and Musculoskeletal and Skin Diseases (NIAMS); National Institute of Diabetes and Digestive and Kidney Diseases (NIDDK); National Institutes of Health (NIH); National Institute of Mental Health (NIMH); Office of Disease Prevention and Health Promotion (ODPHP); Office on Women's Health (OWH); U.S. Department of Agriculture (USDA); U.S. Department of Health and Human Services (HHS); and the U.S. Food and Drug Administration (FDA).

In addition, this volume contains copyrighted documents from the following organizations: National Eating Disorders Association; The Nemours Foundation; and We Are Diabetes.

It may also contain original material produced by Omnigraphics and reviewed by medical consultants.

The photograph on the front cover is © Highwaystarz-Photography/iStock.

Medical Review

Omnigraphics contracts with a team of qualified, senior medical professionals who serve as medical consultants for the *Teen Health Series*. As necessary, medical consultants review reprinted and originally written material for currency and accuracy. Citations including the phrase, Reviewed (month, year)" indicate material reviewed by this team. Medical consultation services are provided to the *Teen Health Series* editors by:

Dr. Vijayalakshmi, MBBS, DGO, MD
Dr. Senthil Selvan, MBBS, DCH, MD
Dr. K. Sivanandham, MBBS, DCH, MS (Research), PhD

About The Teen Health Series

At the request of librarians serving today's young adults, the *Teen Health Series* was developed as a specially focused set of volumes within Omnigraphics' *Health Reference Series*. Each volume deals comprehensively with a topic selected according to the needs and interests of people in middle school and high school. Teens seeking preventive guidance, information about disease warning signs, medical statistics, and risk factors for health problems will find answers to their questions in the *Teen Health Series*. The *Series*, however, is not intended to serve as a tool for diagnosing illness, in prescribing treatments, or as a substitute for the physician/patient relationship. All people concerned about medical symptoms or the possibility of disease are encouraged to seek professional care from an appropriate healthcare provider.

If there is a topic you would like to see addressed in a future volume of the *Teen Health Series*, please write to:

Editor
Teen Health Series
Omnigraphics
615 Griswold, Ste. 901
Detroit, MI 48226

A Note About Spelling And Style

Teen Health Series editors use *Stedman's Medical Dictionary* as an authority for questions related to the spelling of medical terms and the *Chicago Manual of Style* for questions related to grammatical structures, punctuation, and other editorial concerns. Consistent adherence is not always possible, however, because the individual volumes within the *Series* include many documents from a wide variety of different producers and copyright holders, and the editor's primary goal is to present material from each source as accurately as is possible following the terms specified by each document's producer. This sometimes means that information in different chapters or sections may follow other guidelines and alternate spelling authorities.

Part One
Eating Disorders And Their Risk Factors

Chapter 1
Facts About Eating Disorders

Eating Disorders

The eating disorders anorexia nervosa, bulimia nervosa, and binge eating disorder, and their variants, all feature serious disturbances in eating behavior and weight regulation. They are associated with a wide range of adverse psychological, physical, and social consequences. A person with an eating disorder may start out just eating smaller or larger amounts of food, but at some point, their urge to eat less or more spirals out of control. Severe distress or concern about body weight or shape, or extreme efforts to manage weight or food intake, also may characterize an eating disorder.

Eating disorders are real, treatable medical illnesses. They frequently coexist with other illnesses such as depression, substance abuse, or anxiety disorders. Other symptoms can become life-threatening if a person does not receive treatment, which is reflected by anorexia being associated with the highest mortality rate of any psychiatric disorder.

Eating disorders affect both genders, although rates among women and girls are 2½ times greater than among men and boys. Eating disorders frequently appear during the teen years or young adulthood but also may develop during childhood or later in life.

Text under the heading "Eating Disorders" is excerpted from "Eating Disorders: About More Than Food," National Institute of Mental Health (NIMH), November 2014; Text under the heading "Eating Disorder Myths" is excerpted from "9 Eating Disorders Myths Busted," National Institute of Mental Health (NIMH), February 27, 2014.

Causes Of Eating Disorders

Although there is no single known cause of eating disorders, several things may contribute to the development of these disorders:

- **Culture.** In the United States extreme thinness is a social and cultural ideal, and women partially define themselves by how physically attractive they are.

- **Personal characteristics.** Feelings of helplessness, worthlessness, and poor self-image often accompany eating disorders.

- **Other emotional disorders.** Other mental health problems, like depression or anxiety, occur along with eating disorders.

- **Stressful events or life changes.** Things like starting a new school or job or being teased and traumatic events like rape can lead to the onset of eating disorders.

- **Biology.** Studies are being done to look at genes, hormones, and chemicals in the brain that may have an effect on the development of, and recovery from eating disorders.

- **Families.** Parents' attitudes about appearance and diet can affect their kids' attitudes. Also, if your mother or sister has bulimia, you are more likely to have it.

(Source: "Body Image," Office on Women's Health (OWH), U.S. Department of Health and Human Services (HHS).)

Types Of Eating Disorders

Anorexia Nervosa

Many people with anorexia nervosa see themselves as overweight, even when they are clearly underweight. Eating, food, and weight control become obsessions. People with anorexia nervosa typically weigh themselves repeatedly, portion food carefully, and eat very small quantities of only certain foods. Some people with anorexia nervosa also may engage in binge eating followed by extreme dieting, excessive exercise, self-induced vomiting, or misuse of laxatives, diuretics, or enemas.

Symptoms of anorexia nervosa include:

- Extremely low body weight

- Severe food restriction

- Relentless pursuit of thinness and unwillingness to maintain a normal or healthy weight

- Intense fear of gaining weight

- Distorted body image and self-esteem that is heavily influenced by perceptions of body weight and shape, or a denial of the seriousness of low body weight

- Lack of menstruation among girls and women.

Some who have anorexia nervosa recover with treatment after only one episode. Others get well but have relapses. Still others have a more chronic, or long-lasting, form of anorexia nervosa, in which their health declines as they battle the illness.

Other symptoms and medical complications may develop over time, including:

- Thinning of the bones (osteopenia or osteoporosis)

- Brittle hair and nails

- Dry and yellowish skin

- Growth of fine hair all over the body (lanugo)

- Mild anemia, muscle wasting, and weakness

- Severe constipation

- Low blood pressure, or slowed breathing and pulse

- Damage to the structure and function of the heart

- Brain damage

- Multi-organ failure

- Drop in internal body temperature, causing a person to feel cold all the time

- Lethargy, sluggishness, or feeling tired all the time

- Infertility

Bulimia Nervosa

People with bulimia nervosa have recurrent and frequent episodes of eating unusually large amounts of food and feel a lack of control over these episodes. This binge eating is followed by behavior that compensates for the overeating such as forced vomiting, excessive use of laxatives or diuretics, fasting, excessive exercise, or a combination of these behaviors.

Unlike anorexia nervosa, people with bulimia nervosa usually maintain what is considered a healthy or normal weight, while some are slightly overweight. But like people with anorexia nervosa, they often fear gaining weight, want desperately to lose weight, and are intensely unhappy with their body size and shape. Usually, bulimic behavior is done secretly because it is often accompanied by feelings of disgust or shame. The binge eating and purging cycle can happen anywhere from several times a week to many times a day.

Other symptoms include:

- Chronically inflamed and sore throat

- Swollen salivary glands in the neck and jaw area

- Worn tooth enamel, and increasingly sensitive and decaying teeth as a result of exposure to stomach acid

- Acid reflux disorder and other gastrointestinal problems

- Intestinal distress and irritation from laxative abuse

- Severe dehydration from purging of fluids

- Electrolyte imbalance—too low or too high levels of sodium, calcium, potassium, and other minerals that can lead to a heart attack or stroke

Binge Eating Disorder

People with binge eating disorder lose control over their eating. Unlike bulimia nervosa, periods of binge eating are not followed by compensatory behaviors like purging, excessive exercise, or fasting. As a result, people with binge eating disorder often are overweight or obese. People with binge eating disorder who are obese are at higher risk for developing cardiovascular disease and high blood pressure. They also experience guilt, shame, and distress about their binge eating, which can lead to more binge eating.

Treatment For Eating Disorders

Typical treatment goals include restoring adequate nutrition, bringing weight to a healthy level, reducing excessive exercise, and stopping binging and purging behaviors. Specific forms of psychotherapy, or talk therapy—including a family-based therapy called the Maudsley approach and cognitive behavioral approaches—have been shown to be useful for treating specific eating disorders. Evidence also suggests that antidepressant medications approved by the U.S. Food and Drug Administration (FDA) may help for bulimia nervosa and also may be effective for treating co-occurring anxiety or depression for other eating disorders.

Treatment plans often are tailored to individual needs and may include one or more of the following:

- Individual, group, or family psychotherapy

- Medical care and monitoring

- Nutritional counseling

- Medications (for example, antidepressants)

Some patients also may need to be hospitalized to treat problems caused by malnutrition or to ensure they eat enough if they are very underweight. Complete recovery is possible.

Eating Disorder Myths

Myth: You can tell by looking at someone that they have an eating disorder.

Eating disorders come in all shapes and sizes. In fact, with the new DSM-5, you can be at normal or overweight and still get a diagnosis of atypical anorexia nervosa if you have lost a lot of weight. Similarly we will learn about binge eating disorders soon, but you don't have to be overweight or obese to have binge eating disorder. It can happen anywhere along the BMI spectrum.

Myth: Eating disorders are a choice.

Eating disorders are illnesses not choices.

Myth: Genes are destiny.

Hereditability for any of these disorders is not 100 percent. If environment didn't matter, heritability would be 100 percent.

Myth: Eating disorders are benign.

So another myth that we need to bust right away is that eating disorders are somehow trivial or benign. They're not.

Myth: Eating disorders are for life.

Data show that eating disorders are not for life—so eating disorders are treatable. Recovery can and does occur every age.

Eating Disorder Facts

- Eating Disorders do not discriminate, they affect males and females, young and old.

- You can't tell by someone's size whether they have an eating disorder.
- Families do not cause eating disorders—they can be patients' best allies in treatment.
- Both genetic and environmental factors influence eating disorders.
- Eating disorders are serious biologically-influenced mental illnesses, not passing fads.
- Complete recovery is possible.

Chapter 2
Identifying Healthy Eating Patterns

As you get older, you're able to start making your own decisions about a lot of things that matter most to you. You may choose your own clothes, music, and friends. You also may be ready to make decisions about your body and health.

Making healthy decisions about what you eat and drink, how active you are, and how much sleep you get is a great place to start.

Did You Know?

About 20 percent of kids between 12 and 19 years old have obesity. But small changes in your eating and physical activity habits may help you reach and stay a healthy weight.

How Does The Body Use Energy?

Your body needs energy to function and grow. Calories from food and drinks give you that energy. Think of food as energy to charge up your battery for the day. Throughout the day, you use energy from the battery to think and move, so you need to eat and drink to stay powered up. Balancing the energy you take in through food and beverages with the energy you use for growth, activity, and daily living is called "energy balance." Energy balance may help you stay a healthy weight.

About This Chapter: Text in this chapter begins with excerpts from "Take Charge Of Your Health: A Guide For Teenagers," National Institute of Diabetes and Digestive and Kidney Diseases (NIDDK), December 2016; Text under the heading "Understanding And Using The Nutrition Facts Label" is excerpted from "Nutrition Facts Label," U.S. Food and Drug Administration (FDA), October 5, 2016.

How Many Calories Does Your Body Need?

Different people need different amounts of calories to be active or stay a healthy weight. The number of calories you need depends on whether you are male or female, your genes, how old you are, your height and weight, whether you are still growing, and how active you are, which may not be the same every day.

How Should You Manage Or Control Your Weight?

Some teens try to lose weight by eating very little; cutting out whole groups of foods like foods with carbohydrates, or carbs; skipping meals; or fasting. These approaches to losing weight could be unhealthy because they may leave out important nutrients your body needs. In fact, unhealthy dieting could get in the way of trying to manage your weight because it may lead to a cycle of eating very little and then overeating because you get too hungry. Unhealthy dieting could also affect your mood and how you grow.

Smoking, making yourself vomit, or using diet pills or laxatives to lose weight may also lead to health problems. If you make yourself vomit, or use diet pills or laxatives to control your weight, you could have signs of a serious eating disorder and should talk with your healthcare professional or another trusted adult right away. If you smoke, which increases your risk of heart disease, cancer, and other health problems, quit smoking as soon as possible.

If you think you need to lose weight, talk with a healthcare professional first. A doctor or dietitian may be able to tell you if you need to lose weight and how to do so in a healthy way.

Choose Healthy Foods And Drinks

Healthy eating involves taking control of how much and what types of food you eat, as well as the beverages you drink. Try to replace foods high in sugar, salt, and unhealthy fats with fruits, vegetables, whole grains, low-fat protein foods, and fat-free or low-fat dairy foods.

Fruits and Vegetables

Make half of your plate fruits and vegetables. Dark green, red, and orange vegetables have high levels of the nutrients you need, like vitamin C, calcium, and fiber. Adding tomato and spinach—or any other available greens that you like—to your sandwich is an easy way to get more veggies in your meal.

Grains

Choose whole grains like whole-wheat bread, brown rice, oatmeal, and whole-grain cereal, instead of refined-grain cereals, white bread, and white rice.

Protein

Power up with low fat or lean meats like turkey or chicken, and other protein-rich foods, such as seafood, egg whites, beans, nuts, and tofu.

Dairy

Build strong bones with fat-free or low-fat milk products. If you can't digest lactose—the sugar in milk that can cause stomach pain or gas—choose lactose-free milk or soy milk with added calcium. Fat-free or low-fat yogurt is also a good source of dairy food.

Healthy Eating Tips

- Try to limit foods like cookies, candy, frozen desserts, chips, and fries, which often have a lot of sugar, unhealthy fat, and salt.
- For a quick snack, try recharging with a pear, apple, or banana; a small bag of baby carrots; or hummus with sliced veggies.
- Don't add sugar to your food and drinks.
- Drink fat-free or low-fat milk and avoid sugary drinks. Soda, energy drinks, sweet tea, and some juices have added sugars, a source of extra calories. The 2015–2020 Dietary Guidelines call for getting less than 10 percent of your daily calories from added sugars.

Fats

Fat is an important part of your diet. Fat helps your body grow and develop, and may even keep your skin and hair healthy. But fats have more calories per gram than protein or carbs, and some are not healthy.

Some fats, such as oils that come from plants and are liquid at room temperature, are better for you than other fats. Foods that contain healthy oils include avocados, olives, nuts, seeds, and seafood such as salmon and tuna fish.

Solid fats such as butter, stick margarine, and lard, are solid at room temperature. These fats often contain saturated and trans fats, which are not healthy for you. Other foods with saturated fats include fatty meats, and cheese and other dairy products made from whole milk. Take it easy on foods like fried chicken, cheeseburgers, and fries, which often have a lot of saturated and trans fats. Options to consider include a turkey sandwich with mustard or a lean-meat, turkey, or veggie burger.

Your body needs a small amount of sodium, which is mostly found in salt. But getting too much sodium from your foods and drinks can raise your blood pressure, which is unhealthy for your heart and your body in general. Even though you're a teen, it's important to pay attention to your blood pressure and heart health now to prevent health problems as you get older.

Try to consume less than 2,300 mg, or no more than 1 teaspoon, of sodium a day. This amount includes the salt in already prepared food, as well as the salt you add when cooking or eating your food.

Processed foods, like those that are canned or packaged, often have more sodium than unprocessed foods, such as fresh fruits and vegetables. When you can, choose fresh or frozen fruits and veggies over processed foods. Try adding herbs and spices instead of salt to season your food if you make your own meals. Remember to rinse canned vegetables with water to remove extra salt. If you use packaged foods, check the amount of sodium listed on the Nutrition Facts Label.

Be Media Smart

Advertisements, television shows, the Internet, and social media may affect your food and beverage choices and how you choose to spend your time. Many ads try to get you to consume high-fat foods and sugary drinks. Be aware of some of the tricks ads use to influence you:

- An ad may show a group of teens consuming a food or drink, or using a product to make you think all teens are or should be doing the same. The ad may even use phrases like "all teens need" or "all teens are."
- Advertisers sometimes show famous people using or recommending a product because they think you will want to buy products that your favorite celebrities use.
- Ads often use cartoon figures to make a food, beverage, or activity look exciting and appealing to young people.

Limit Added Sugars

Some foods, like fruit, are naturally sweet. Other foods, like ice cream and baked desserts, as well as some beverages, have added sugars to make them taste sweet. These sugars add calories but not vitamins or fiber. Try to consume less than 10 percent of your daily calories from added sugars in food and beverages. Reach for an apple or banana instead of a candy bar.

Did You Know?

Many teens need more of these nutrients:

- Calcium, to build strong bones and teeth. Good sources of calcium are fat-free or low-fat milk, yogurt, and cheese.

- Vitamin D, to keep bones healthy. Good sources of vitamin D include orange juice, whole oranges, tuna, and fat-free or low-fat milk.
- Potassium, to help lower blood pressure. Try a banana, or baked potato with the skin, for a potassium boost.
- Fiber, to help you stay regular and feel full. Good sources of fiber include beans and celery.
- Protein, to power you up and help you grow strong. Peanut butter; eggs; tofu; legumes, such as lentils and peas; and chicken, fish, and low-fat meats are all good sources of protein.
- Iron, to help you grow. Red meat contains a form of iron that your body absorbs best. Spinach, beans, peas, and iron-fortified cereals are also sources of iron. You can help your body absorb the iron from these foods better when you also eat foods with vitamin C, like an orange.

Control Your Food Portions

A portion is how much food or beverage you choose to consume at one time, whether in a restaurant, from a package, at school or a friend's, or at home. Many people consume larger portions than they need, especially when away from home. Ready-to-eat meals—from a restaurant, grocery store, or at school—may give you larger portions than your body needs to stay charged up. The Weight-control Information Network has tips to help you eat and drink a suitable amount of food and beverages for you, whether you are at home or somewhere else.

Did You Know?

Just one super-sized, fast food meal may have more calories than you need in a whole day. And when people are served more food, they may eat or drink more—even if they don't need it. This habit may lead to weight gain. When consuming fast food, choose small portions or healthier options, like a veggie wrap or salad instead of fries or fried chicken.

Don't Skip Meals

Skipping meals might seem like an easy way to lose weight, but it actually may lead to weight gain if you eat more later to make up for it. Even if you're really busy with school and activities, it's important to try not to skip meals.

Follow these tips to keep your body charged up all day and to stay healthy:

- **Eat breakfast every day.** Breakfast helps your body get going. If you're short on time in the morning, grab something to go, like an apple or banana.

- **Pack your lunch on school days.** Packing your lunch may help you control your food and beverage portions and increases the chances that you will eat it because you made it.

- **Eat dinner with your family.** When you eat home-cooked meals with your family, you are more likely to consume healthy foods. Having meals together also gives you a chance to reconnect with each other and share news about your day.

- **Get involved in grocery shopping and meal planning at home.** Going food shopping and planning and preparing meals with family members or friends can be fun. Not only can you choose a favorite grocery store, and healthy foods and recipes, you also have a chance to help others in your family eat healthy too.

10 Tips: Eating Foods Away From Home

Restaurants, convenience and grocery stores, or fast-food places offer a variety of options when eating out. But larger portions can make it easy to eat or drink too many calories. Larger helpings can also increase your intake of saturated fat, sodium, and added sugars. Think about ways to make healthier choices when eating food away from home.

1. **Consider your drink**

   Choose water, fat-free or low-fat milk, unsweetened tea, and other drinks without added sugars to complement your meal.

2. **Savor a salad**

   Start your meal with a salad packed with vegetables to help you feel satisfied sooner. Ask for dressing on the side and use a small amount of it.

3. **Share a main dish**

   Divide a main entree between family and friends. Ask for small plates for everyone at the table.

4. **Select from the sides**

   Order a side dish or an appetizer-sized portion instead of a regular entree. They're usually served on smaller plates and in smaller amounts.

5. Pack your snack

Pack fruit, sliced vegetables, low-fat string cheese, or unsalted nuts to eat during road trips or long commutes. No need to stop for other food when these snacks are ready-to-eat.

6. Fill your plate with vegetables and fruit

Stir-fries, kabobs, or vegetarian menu items usually have more vegetables. Select fruits as a side dish or dessert.

7. Compare the calories, fat, and sodium

Many menus now include nutrition information. Look for items that are lower in calories, saturated fat, and sodium. Check with your server if you don't see them on the menu. For more information, check the U.S. Food and Drug Administration's (FDA) website.

8. Pass on the buffet

Have an item from the menu and avoid the "all-you-can-eat" buffet. Steamed, grilled, or broiled dishes have fewer calories than foods that are fried in oil or cooked in butter.

9. Get your whole grains

Request 100 percent whole-wheat breads, rolls, and pasta when choosing sandwiches, burgers, or main dishes.

10. Quit the "clean your plate" club

Decide to save some for another meal. Take leftovers home in a container and chill in the refrigerator right away.

(Source: "10 Tips: Eating Foods Away from Home," United States Department of Agriculture (USDA).)

Planning Healthy Meals And Physical Activities Just For You

Being healthy sounds like it could be a lot of work, right? Well, it doesn't have to be. A free, online tool called the MyPlate Daily Checklist can help you create a daily food plan. All you have to do is type in whether you are male or female, your weight, height, and how much physical activity you get each day. The checklist will tell you how many daily calories you should take in and what amounts of fruit, vegetables, grains, protein, and dairy you should eat to stay within your calorie target.

Another tool, called the SuperTracker, can help you plan, analyze, and track both your eating patterns and physical activity. With SuperTracker, you can find out what and how much to eat, track your foods, physical activities and weight, and set personal goals.

With SuperTracker's Food-A-Pedia, you can type in a food or beverage to find out how many calories it has, as well as how much sugar, saturated fat, and sodium. The tool has nutrition information for more than 8,000 foods. You can use Food-A-Pedia to plan meals like the ones below:

Breakfast: A banana, a slice of whole-grain bread with avocado or tomato, and fat-free or low-fat milk.

Lunch: A turkey sandwich with dark leafy lettuce, tomato, and red peppers on whole-wheat bread.

Dinner: Two whole-grain taco shells with chicken or black beans, fat-free or low-fat cheese, and romaine lettuce.

Snack: An apple, banana, or air-popped popcorn.

Be A Health Champion

Spending much of your day away from home can sometimes make it hard to consume healthy foods and drinks. By becoming a "health champion," you can help yourself and family members, as well as your friends, get healthier by consuming healthier foods and drinks and becoming more active. Use the checklist below to work healthy habits into your day, whether you're at home or on the go.

Tips To Follow

- Each night, pack a healthy lunch and snacks for the next day. Consume the lunch you packed. Try to avoid soda, chips, and candy from vending machines.
- Go to bed at a regular time every night to recharge your body and mind. Turn off your phone, television, and other devices when you go to bed. Try to get between 8 and 10 hours of sleep each night.
- Eat a healthy breakfast.
- Walk or bike to school if you live nearby and can do so safely. Invite friends to join you.
- Between classes, stand up and walk around, even if your next subject is in the same room.
- Participate in gym classes instead of sitting on the sidelines.
- Get involved in choosing food and drinks at home. Help make dinner and share it with your family at the dinner table.

Understanding And Using The Nutrition Facts Label

The Nutrition Facts Label found on packaged foods and beverages is your daily tool for making informed food choices that contribute to healthy lifelong eating habits. Figure. 2.1. below shows an updated food label, which the U.S. Food and Drug Administration (FDA) has approved for use on most packaged foods beginning in 2018. Explore it and discover the wealth of information it contains!

Nutrition Facts

8 servings per container

Serving size   **2/3 cup (55g)**

Amount per serving

Calories   230

% Daily Value*

Total Fat 8g	**10%**
Saturated Fat 1g	**5%**
Trans Fat 0g	
Cholesterol 0mg	**0%**
Sodium 160mg	**7%**
Total Carbohydrate 37g	**13%**
Dietary Fiber 4g	**14%**
Total Sugars 12g	
Includes 10g Added Sugars	**20%**
Protein 3g	
Vitamin D 2mcg	10%
Calcium 260mg	20%
Iron 8mg	45%
Potassium 235mg	6%

* The % Daily Value (DV) tells you how much a nutrient in a serving of food contributes to a daily diet. 2,000 calories a day is used for general nutrition advice.

Figure. 2.1. Nutrition Facts Label

- **Serving Size** is based on **the amount of food that is customarily eaten** at one time. All of the nutrition information listed on the Nutrition Facts Label is based on **one serving** of the food.

- When comparing calories and nutrients in different foods, check the serving size in order to make an accurate comparison.

- **Servings Per Container** shows the **total number of servings** in the entire food package or container. One package of food may contain more than one serving.

- If a package contains *two servings* and you eat the entire package, you have consumed *twice the amount of calories and nutrients* listed on the label.

- **Calories** refers to the **total number of calories,** or "energy," supplied from all sources (fat, carbohydrate, protein, and alcohol) in one serving of the food.

- To achieve or maintain a healthy weight, balance the number of calories you consume with the number of calories your body uses.

As a general rule:

- **100 calories** per serving is **moderate**

- **400 calories** per serving is **high**

- **Calories from Fat** are *not* additional calories, but are **fat's contribution to the total number of calories** in one serving of the food.

- "Fat-free" doesn't mean "calorie-free." Some lower fat food items may have as many calories as the full-fat versions.

The Nutrition Facts Label can help you learn about the nutrient content of many foods in your diet. It enables you to monitor the nutrients you want to get less of and those you want to get more of.

- **Nutrients to get less of**—get less than 100 percent DV of these nutrients each day: saturated fat, trans fat, cholesterol, and sodium. (Note: trans fat has no %DV, so use the amount of grams as a guide.)

- **Nutrients to get more of**—get 100 percent DV of these nutrients on most days: dietary fiber, vitamin A, vitamin C, calcium, and iron.

- **% Daily Value** (%DV) shows **how much of a nutrient** is in one serving of the food. The %DV column doesn't add up vertically to 100 percent. Instead, the %DV is the percentage of the Daily Value (the amounts of key nutrients recommended per day for Americans 4 years of age and older) for each nutrient in one serving of the food.

- Use the %DV to compare food products and to choose products that are higher in nutrients you want to get more of and lower in nutrients you want to get less of.

As a general rule:

- **5 percent DV** or less of a nutrient per serving is **low**

- **20 percent DV** or more of a nutrient per serving is **high**

- **Footnote with Daily Values**

Some of the %DVs are based on a **2,000 calorie daily diet**. However, your Daily Values may be higher or lower depending on your calorie needs, which vary according to age, gender, height, weight, and physical activity level.

- If there is enough space available on the food package, the Nutrition Facts Label will also list the **Daily Values** and **goals** for some key nutrients. These are given for both a 2,000 and 2,500 calorie daily diet.

Chapter 3
Causes And Risk Factors For Eating Disorders

Eating disorders involve extreme emotions, attitudes, and behaviors involving weight and food. The most common eating disorders include:

- Anorexia Nervosa

- Binge Eating

- Bulimia

Risk Factors For Eating Disorders

Eating disorders are more than just a problem with food. Food is used to feel in control of other feelings that may seem overwhelming. For example, starving is a way for people with anorexia to feel more in control of their lives and to ease tension, anger, and anxiety. Purging and other behaviors to prevent weight gain are ways for people with bulimia to feel more in control of their lives and to ease stress and anxiety.

Although there is no single known cause of eating disorders, several things may contribute to the development of these disorders:

- **Culture.** In the United States extreme thinness is a social and cultural ideal, and women partially define themselves by how physically attractive they are.
- **Personal characteristics.** Feelings of helplessness, worthlessness, and poor self-image often accompany eating disorders.
- **Other emotional disorders.** Other mental health problems, like depression or anxiety, occur along with eating disorders.

About This Chapter: This chapter includes text excerpted from "Eating Disorders," MentalHealth.gov, U.S. Department of Health and Human Services (HHS), April 26, 2016.

- **Stressful events or life changes.** Things like starting a new school or job or being teased and traumatic events like rape can lead to the onset of eating disorders.
- **Biology.** Studies are being done to look at genes, hormones, and chemicals in the brain that may have an effect on the development of, and recovery from eating disorders.
- **Families.** Parents' attitudes about appearance and diet can affect their kids' attitudes. Also, if your mother or sister has bulimia, you are more likely to have it.

(Source: "Body Image," Office on Women's Health (OWH).)

Anorexia Nervosa

Anorexia nervosa is an eating disorder that makes people lose more weight than is considered healthy for their age and height.

Persons with this disorder may have an intense fear of weight gain, even when they are underweight. They may diet or exercise too much, or use other methods to lose weight.

Causes

The exact causes of anorexia nervosa are not known. Many factors probably are involved. Genes and hormones may play a role. Social attitudes that promote very thin body types may also be involved.

Family conflicts are no longer thought to contribute to this or other eating disorders.

Risk factors for anorexia include:

- Being more worried about, or paying more attention to, weight and shape
- Having an anxiety disorder as a child
- Having a negative self-image
- Having eating problems during infancy or early childhood
- Having certain social or cultural ideas about health and beauty
- Trying to be perfect or overly focused on rules

Anorexia usually begins during the teen years or young adulthood. It is more common in females, but may also be seen in males. The disorder is seen mainly in white women who are high academic achievers and who have a goal-oriented family or personality.

Symptoms

To be diagnosed with anorexia, a person must:

- Have an intense fear of gaining weight or becoming fat, even when she is underweight
- Refuse to keep weight at what is considered normal for her age and height (15 percent or more below the normal weight)
- Have a body image that is very distorted, be very focused on body weight or shape, and refuse to admit the seriousness of weight loss
- Have not had a period for three or more cycles (in women)

People with anorexia may severely limit the amount of food they eat, or eat and then make themselves throw up. Other behaviors include:

- Cutting food into small pieces or moving them around the plate instead of eating
- Exercising all the time, even when the weather is bad, they are hurt, or their schedule is busy
- Going to the bathroom right after meals
- Refusing to eat around other people
- Using pills to make themselves urinate (water pills or diuretics), have a bowel movement (enemas and laxatives), or decrease their appetite (diet pills)

Other symptoms of anorexia may include:

- Blotchy or yellow skin that is dry and covered with fine hair
- Confused or slow thinking, along with poor memory or judgment
- Depression
- Dry mouth
- Extreme sensitivity to cold (wearing several layers of clothing to stay warm)
- Loss of bone strength
- Wasting away of muscle and loss of body fat

Binge Eating

Binge eating is when a person eats a much larger amount of food in a shorter period of time than he or she normally would. During binge eating, the person also feels a loss of control.

Considerations

A binge eater often:

- Eats 5,000–15,000 calories in one sitting
- Often snacks, in addition to eating three meals a day
- Overeats throughout the day

Binge eating by itself usually leads to becoming overweight.

Binge eating may occur on its own or with another eating disorder, such as bulimia. People with bulimia typically eat large amounts of high-calorie foods, usually in secret. After this binge eating they often force themselves to vomit or take laxatives.

Causes

The cause of binge eating is unknown. However, binge eating often begins during or after strict dieting.

Bulimia

Bulimia is an illness in which a person binges on food or has regular episodes of overeating and feels a loss of control. The person then uses different methods—such as vomiting or abusing laxatives—to prevent weight gain.

Many (but not all) people with bulimia also have anorexia nervosa.

Causes

Many more women than men have bulimia. The disorder is most common in adolescent girls and young women. The affected person is usually aware that her eating pattern is abnormal and may feel fear or guilt with the binge purge episodes.

The exact cause of bulimia is unknown. Genetic, psychological, trauma, family, society, or cultural factors may play a role. Bulimia is likely due to more than one factor.

Symptoms

In bulimia, eating binges may occur as often as several times a day for many months.

People with bulimia often eat large amounts of high-calorie foods, usually in secret. People can feel a lack of control over their eating during these episodes.

Binges lead to self-disgust, which causes purging to prevent weight gain. Purging may include:

- Forcing yourself to vomit

- Excessive exercise

- Using laxatives, enemas, or diuretics (water pills)

Purging often brings a sense of relief.

People with bulimia are often at a normal weight, but they may see themselves as being overweight. Because the person's weight is often normal, other people may not notice this eating disorder.

Symptoms that other people can see include:

- Compulsive exercise

- Suddenly eating large amounts of food or buying large amounts of food that disappear right away

- Regularly going to the bathroom right after meals

- Throwing away packages of laxatives, diet pills, emetics (drugs that cause vomiting), or diuretics

Health Risks

Anorexia nervosa. Anorexia can slow the heart rate and lower blood pressure, increasing the chance of heart failure. Those who use drugs to stimulate vomiting, bowel movements, or urination are also at high risk for heart failure. Starvation can also lead to heart failure, as well as damage the brain. Anorexia may also cause hair and nails to grow brittle. Skin may dry out, become yellow, and develop a covering of soft hair called lanugo. Mild anemia, swollen joints, reduced muscle mass, and light-headedness also commonly occur as a consequence of this eating disorder. Severe cases of anorexia can lead to brittle bones that break easily as a result of calcium loss.

Binge-eating disorder. Binge-eating disorder can cause high blood pressure and high cholesterol levels. Other effects of binge-eating disorder include fatigue, joint pain, Type II diabetes, gallbladder disease, and heart disease.

Bulimia nervosa. The acid in vomit can wear down the outer layer of the teeth, inflame and damage the esophagus (a tube in the throat through which food passes to the stomach), and enlarge the glands near the cheeks (giving the appearance of swollen cheeks). Damage to the stomach can also occur from frequent vomiting. Irregular heartbeats, heart failure, and death can occur from chemical imbalances and the loss of important minerals such as potassium. Peptic ulcers, pancreatitis (inflammation of the pancreas, which is a large gland that aids digestion), and long-term constipation are also consequences of bulimia.

(Source: "Eating Disorders," Substance Abuse and Mental Health Service Administration (SAMHSA).)

Chapter 4

Eating Disorders—Not Just A Women's Issue

Men And Body Image Issues

Did you know that men, like women, can struggle with body image issues or an eating disorder? Men may feel a lot of pressure to have a "perfect," muscular body and may focus too much on exercise and dieting. This focus can wind up hurting a man's body, job, and relationships. But medicines and counseling can help men with eating and body image disorders lead healthy lives.

Signs And Symptoms Of Eating Disorder

- Eating tiny portions, refusing to eat, and denying hunger
- Dressing in loose, baggy clothing (to hide weight loss)
- Exercising excessively and compulsively
- Feeling cold frequently Experiencing hair loss, sunken eyes, or pale skin Complaining of being fat, even when underweight
- Developing lanugo, fine body hair that develops along the midsection, legs, and arms
- Eating little in public but overeating in private
- Disappearing after eating; spending a lot of time in the bathroom

---

About This Chapter: This chapter includes text excerpted from "Mental Health For Men," Office on Women's Health (OWH), U.S. Department of Health and Human Services (HHS), January 10, 2011. Reviewed March 2017.

- Experiencing severe dental problems (loss of enamel)
- Hiding food to eat later Eating little in public but overeating in private
- Hiding food wrappers and other evidence of binge eating

(Source: "Clients With Substance Abuse And Eating Disorders," Substance Abuse and Mental Health Services Administration (SAMHSA).)

Eating Disorders

Eating disorders involve extreme emotions, attitudes, and behaviors around weight and food. The most common eating disorder for men is binge eating disorder.

With binge eating disorder, people eat a lot of food even if they feel full. They sometimes may try to make up for their overeating episodes by dieting. Other eating disorders that affect men include anorexia and bulimia.

Muscle Mistakes

Some men try to pump up their muscles by taking anabolic steroids. But using steroids in this way can harm your physical and mental health—and it's illegal. Also, injecting steroids raises your risk of getting human immunodeficiency virus (HIV) and hepatitis.

Sometimes, men try natural supplements like creatine to build muscle. Keep in mind that "natural" doesn't necessarily mean safe. Make sure to discuss any supplements with your doctor before taking them.

Body Image Issues

People with body image issues may feel unhappy with how they look and feel self-conscious about their bodies. If these feelings are extreme, the person may have body dysmorphic disorder (BDD). People with BDD have extreme concern over what they see as flaws. Men and women are affected equally but may focus on different parts of the body. Men tend to worry more about their skin, hair, nose, muscles, and genitals.

Obsession with food or how you look can be very painful. If you have eating or body image issues, don't let shame or embarrassment keep you from seeking help.

Mental Health For Men

Mental health helps us face the challenges in our life, makes us feel comfortable, supports our physical health, and more. But day-to-day stress and difficult times can wear down our mental health. Major changes like losing a job, the death of a loved one, going off to combat or coming out as gay can be especially hard. And even happy times—like becoming a father—can take a toll on your emotions.

Today, we know a lot more about ways to promote mental health. Try some simple steps, like making sure to get enough sleep, getting social support, exercising, and finding healthy ways to cope when you feel stressed.

If you are struggling with your mental health, you are not alone. In fact, about 1 out of 4 American adults suffers from a mental health condition each year. Experts don't know exactly what causes mental illnesses, but a combination of genes and life events often is involved. It's important to remember that mental health disorders are real medical illnesses that can't be willed or wished away.

Chapter 5
Eating Disorders: What To Watch For

Eating disorders or disordered eating includes anorexia nervosa, bulimia nervosa, and other disorders. While most people struggling with an eating disorder show behaviors that don't fit cleanly into any one disease definition, here are the basic definitions:

- Anorexia nervosa is when a person restricts how much they eat, leading to low body weight as well as a fear of gaining weight or becoming fat. People with anorexia also judge themselves largely on their weight or body shape and don't recognize the seriousness of their own low body weight.

- Bulimia nervosa, in general, is defined as recurrent episodes of binge eating followed by some inappropriate behavior to compensate for these episodes, such as vomiting or taking laxatives. People with bulimia also judge themselves largely on their weight or body shape.

- Binge eating is eating more food at one time than most people would, because a person feels a loss of control of his or her ability to stop eating.

Eating disorders are common. While estimates vary widely, one study suggested that approximately 1 in every 4 high school girls has symptoms of an eating disorder. The same study suggested that about 1 in 10 boys has symptoms, too. Genetics play a role, and there are other factors that put girls at risk for eating disorders. Participation in activities where being thin is considered helpful, such as dancing, gymnastics, modeling, and running, puts people at higher risk for developing eating disorders. People who diet are also at higher risk.

About This Chapter: This chapter includes text excerpted from "Eating Disorders: What To Watch For," Office on Women's Health (OWH), U.S. Department of Health and Human Services (HHS), February 28, 2017.

What can you do to help identify an eating disorder in yourself or others? First, look out for these signs:

- Having a lot of concern or an obsession about weight and food

- Being very defensive about eating or weight loss habits

- Having a fear of food, or changing plans to avoid eating

- Exercising excessively

- Losing weight or not gaining weight when still growing taller (ask your doctor about how your weight should be changing, if at all)

- Going on extremely restrictive diets

- Eating large amounts of food at once (binge eating)

- Vomiting or using diuretics, laxatives, diet pills, stimulants, steroids, or ipecac

- Involvement or interest with pro-anorexia or pro-bulimia websites (yes, they exist)

- Not having regular periods

- Feeling weak, faint, or dizzy, bruising easily, looking pale, complaining of being cold a lot, losing your hair, or having abdominal pain

- Not hanging out with friends during mealtimes

- Experiencing mood changes or depression

- Growing thin, soft hair on your body's midsection and extremities

- Having cavities or erosion of the enamel on your teeth

If you notice any of these symptoms in yourself, make sure that you tell an adult you trust (if you are a teen) and see a doctor or nurse as soon as possible. Make sure that the doctor screens you for eating disorders by telling them that you are concerned about an eating disorder. If you see these symptoms in a friend or family member, please talk to them privately and express concern for them. Offer your support and offer to go to a doctor with them. Don't blame them for their behavior. If you are still concerned after speaking with them, speak to a trusted medical professional, adult, school counselor, or parent for help. You won't be able to fix this problem by yourself. Your friend will need to get the help of a doctor or counselor. Also, follow up with your friend or family member and make sure they are getting help.

A Personal Story

By Dr. Alan E. Simon, M.D., Medical Officer, Office on Women's Health

When I was a teenager, during the long winter month of February, I would often look forward to the warm weather and getting back to summer camp. Being a summer camp counselor was the best part of the year. But now that I am a pediatrician, I often think back on summer camp and remember one thing that I wish I had done differently.

When I was a counselor-in-training, Molly*, one of my close friends at summer camp, was the person that all the other campers and counselors wanted to be around. She had endless patience with the campers and shared at least one inside joke with every counselor. She smiled almost all of the time, and, although she was a little overweight, Molly was a talented athlete who was often tasked to teach basketball, volleyball, and swimming.

One year when Molly and I were both junior counselors, she looked different. She retained her ever-present smile, and she had also dropped a lot of weight. She looked healthy and happy, and everyone told her so.

But by the next summer, Molly had lost more weight. A lot more weight. Only, she didn't look healthy or happy this year. Even as teenagers in the 80's, we'd heard of eating disorders and suspected that she had one, but none of us really knew what to do or what to say to her... so we said nothing. If I could go back, I would have intervened, armed with the knowledge I have now.

I still see Molly every now and again, and I think about how lucky she was. One in 20 people with anorexia nervosa and about 1 in 25 people with bulimia nervosa die from the disease. As a pediatrician, I have seen teenagers who are dangerously sick from their eating disorders. Eating disorders can cause problems with any body system, including heart problems and kidney problems. Fortunately, after that summer, Molly did seek treatment, and she has been at a healthy weight for a very long time. When I see her now, she reminds me of the happy Molly I met that first summer.

Name changed to preserve confidentiality.

Chapter 6

Negative Body Image May Contribute To Eating Disorders

Do you wish you could lose weight, get taller, or develop faster? It's pretty common to worry a little about how your body looks, especially when it's changing. You can learn about body image and ways to take control of yours.

What Is Body Image?

Body image is how you think and feel about your body. It includes whether you think you look good to other people.

Body image is affected by a lot of things, including messages you get from your friends, family, and the world around you. Images we see in the media definitely affect our body image even though a lot of media images are changed or aren't realistic.

Why does body image matter? Your body image can affect how you feel about yourself overall. For example, if you are unhappy with your looks, your self-esteem may start to go down. Sometimes, having body image issues or low self-esteem may lead to depression, eating disorders, or obesity.

Stressing About Body Changes

During puberty and your teen years, your body changes a lot. All those changes can be hard to handle. They might make you worry about what other people think of how you look and about whether your body is normal. If you have these kinds of concerns, you are not alone.

About This Chapter: This chapter includes text excerpted from "Having Body Image Issues," GirlsHealth.gov, Office on Women's Health (OWH), January 7, 2015.

Here are some common thoughts about changing bodies.

- Why am I taller than most of the boys my age?

- Why haven't I grown?

- Am I too skinny?

- Am I too fat?

- Will others like me now that I am changing?

- Are my breasts too small?

- Are my breasts too large?

- Why do I have acne?

- Do my clothes look right on my body?

- Are my hips getting bigger?

If you are stressed about your body, you may feel better if you understand why you are changing so fast—or not changing as fast as your friends.

During puberty, you get taller and see other changes in your body, such as wider hips and thighs. Your body will also start to have more fat compared to muscle than before. Each young woman changes at her own pace, and all of these changes are normal.

Want to know more about how your body and mind may be changing? You can read all about puberty. You also can work on feeling good about your body while it's changing.

What Are Serious Body Image Problems?

If how your body looks bothers you a lot and you can't stop thinking about it, you could have body dysmorphic disorder, or BDD.

People with BDD think they look ugly even if they have a small flaw or none at all. They may spend many hours a day looking at flaws and trying to hide them. They also may ask friends to reassure them about their looks or want to have a lot of cosmetic surgery. If you or a friend may have BDD, talk to an adult you trust, such as a parent or guardian, school counselor, teacher, doctor, or nurse. BDD is an illness, and you can get help.

Chapter 7

Genetics And The Impact Of Culture On Eating Disorders

Genetics And Eating Disorder

The presence of eating disorders tends to be influenced by hereditary within families, with female relatives most often diagnosed. This hereditary component may suggest that there is a genetic component as well as environmental elements to the disorder onset. In terms of the latter, the environmental factors that could be causes of an eating disorder include the social pressure to be thin, high social class, high social anxiety, elevated weight or obesity, high impulsivity, individual differences in biological response to starvation, and individual differences in the reward value of starvation or eating.

It is important to recognize that a genetic component may play a role in people struggling with disordered eating, particularly since the diagnosis of anorexia nervosa (AN) is currently based solely on signs and symptoms as opposed to objective measures. The criteria of AN remains the subject of considerable debate, in large part because it fails to result in clearly defined subgroups or to account for changing symptomatology over the course of the illness. Many individuals who suffer from disordered eating do not meet the criteria for AN and bulimia nervosa, so they are placed in a residual group known as eating disorder not otherwise specified. It was stated that risk-factor studies that include both the genetic and environmental factors present an untapped source of information of potential value for revising the current classification system.

About This Chapter: Text under the heading "Genetics And Eating Disorder" is excerpted from "Coming Together to Calm the Hunger: Group Therapy Program for Adults Diagnosed with Anorexia Nervosa," U.S. Department of Education (ED), March 4, 2012. Reviewed March 2017; Text under the heading "Other Environmental And Cultural Factors," is excerpted from "Environmental Factors in Eating Disorder Development," © 2017 Omnigraphics, Reviewed March 2017.

Understanding the genetic components of AN is valuable for treatment. Treatment is best accomplished when the causes of a disorder are known as this aids in the search for effective interventions. It is interesting to note that some individuals with a family history of AN do not develop AN, whereas others will develop disordered eating; it has been asserted that this is a gene plus an environmental interaction whereby varying genotypes would render individuals differentially sensitive to environmental events.

An excellent example of this was provided where an individual with Genotype A might experiment with her first extreme diet, find the experience aversive and uncomfortable, and reject the behavior on the basis of it not being at all reinforcing. In contrast, an individual with Genotype B might experience that first episode of severe caloric restriction to be highly reinforcing by reducing her innate dysphoria and anxiety, providing her with a sense of control over her own body weight and resulting in her receiving positive social attention for weight-loss attempts.

Identification of risk factors is important for determining high-risk groups for targeted interventions, designing prevention program content, and informing public policy.

Other Environmental And Cultural Factors

Researchers cannot pinpoint a single cause for eating disorders. Instead, they view eating disorders as complex illnesses that can have a variety of contributing causes, including genetic, biological, psychological, social, and environmental factors. Some of the environmental factors that may increase the likelihood of an individual developing an eating disorder include sociocultural pressures to attain a certain standard of thinness, media messages about diet and weight loss, exposure to traumatic events, stressful or chaotic family dynamics, and mothers who frequently express dissatisfaction with their own bodies or criticize their daughters' body shape or weight.

Sociocultural Ideals

American media and popular culture promote an image of the ideal or "perfect" body that is unattainable for most people. Fashion models, actors, and celebrities featured onscreen or in magazines tend to fall within a narrow set of norms that include only those who are extremely thin or extremely muscular, and editing technologies such as Photoshop and airbrushing are often employed to remove any blemishes, wrinkles, or love handles. When people internalize these unrealistic standards of beauty, it may contribute to the development of a negative body image, an obsession with weight and appearance, and eating disorders. Although many people who are exposed to sociocultural ideals of thinness do not develop eating disorders, studies have shown that some individuals are highly vulnerable to such environmental messages about weight and beauty.

Dieting

In response to societal pressures to attain a certain ideal body shape, many people resort to restrictive dieting or other extreme weight-loss measures. Americans spend an estimated $60 billion each year on fad diets and dangerous weight-loss products, despite the fact that 95 percent of people on diets fail to achieve permanent weight loss. In addition to their ineffectiveness, restrictive diets are also a common precipitating factor in the development of eating disorders. Dieting increases people's preoccupation with food and weight and generates feelings of guilt and shame surrounding eating. For some people, these feelings contribute to the development of eating disorders.

Traumatic Experiences

Studies have suggested that up to 50 percent of people with eating disorders have experienced a traumatic event, such as physical or sexual abuse. Such events often create feelings of guilt and shame and contribute to a negative body image. Some victims of trauma develop eating disorders as they restrict food in an attempt to regain control over their bodies or cope with the intense emotions generated by the event.

Family Dynamics

Stressful or chaotic family situations are another environmental factor that has been linked with an increase in the likelihood of eating disorders. While many people with eating disorders come from difficult family environments, however, there is no evidence to support the idea that certain family situations or parenting styles directly cause eating disorders. Instead, family dynamics are only one factor that may potentially contribute to the illness. In addition, research has found that the relationship may be reciprocal—the stress surrounding a member's struggle with an eating disorder may cause negative family dynamics to develop.

On the other hand, family support systems can also help young people ignore sociocultural pressures and establish a positive body image, which may help protect them from developing eating disorders.

Finally, family involvement is a vital component in the treatment and recovery process.

The Mother-Daughter Relationship

Of all the family relationships, the one between mothers and daughters has been most extensively studied with respect to its impact on the development of eating disorders. Research has suggested a correlation between a mother's body image and eating behaviors and the likelihood of her daughter developing an eating disorder. Some of this the correlation may be explained by genetic predisposition, which is estimated to account for between 50 and 80 percent of eating disorder risk, yet many experts believe that behavior modeling also plays a role.

Studies have identified the following behaviors by mothers as factors that may increase the risk of daughters developing low self-esteem, negative body image, preoccupation with weight and appearance, and eating disorders:

- Mothers who have a negative body image or frequently express dissatisfaction with their own weight, shape, or size;

- Mothers who have disordered eating habits and attitudes, such as restrictive dieting or binge eating;

- Mothers who criticize or ridicule their daughters' food choices or eating habits;

- Mothers who make negative comments about their daughters' weight and appearance;

- Mothers who insist upon a relationship with their daughters that lacks boundaries and does not promote individual autonomy.

It is important to note that eating disorders never have a single cause. Even if mothers engage in one or more of the above behaviors, they should not be blamed for having a daughter with an eating disorder. But being aware of the risks associated with the mother-daughter relationship can help people adjust their behavior and build healthier family dynamics. Mothers who focus on health and inner beauty rather than weight and appearance can help counteract other environmental factors and protect their daughters against disordered eating behaviors.

References

1. Fielder-Jenks, Chelsea. "Mothers, Daughters, and Eating Disorders," Eating Disorder Hope, 2016.

2. Jones, Megan. "Factors that May Contribute to Eating Disorders," National Eating Disorders Association, n.d.

Chapter 8
Media And Eating Disorders

Weight Bias[1]

Weight bias can be defined as the inclination to form unreasonable judgments based on a person's weight. Stigma is the social sign that is carried by a person who is a victim of prejudice and weight bias. Obese children are at an increased risk for bias as a result of their weight.

Weight bias is caused by a general belief that stigma and shame will motivate people to lose weight or the belief that people fail to lose weight as a result of inadequate self-discipline or insufficient willpower. Our culture may not punish people who practice weight bias because our culture values thinness. Society frequently blames the victim rather than addressing environmental conditions that contribute to obesity.

Weight bias affects the child in multiple ways. Obese children are often the brunt of teasing or discrimination. Bias exists in the adult workplace and may affect children as they enter the workforce. Weight bias also influences educational success and may affect how healthcare is delivered. Weight bias is promoted in the media and even by parents of obese children. Curbing the obesity epidemic will require new strategies that do not result in bias or prejudice.

This chapter includes text excerpted from documents published by two public domain sources. Text in this chapter begins with the heading marked 1 is excerpted from "Childhood Obesity: Issues Of Weight Bias," Centers for Disease Control and Prevention (CDC), March 30, 2012. Reviewed March 2017; Text under headings marked 2 are excerpted from "Media-Smart Youth: Eat, Think, And Be Active!" *Eunice Kennedy Shriver* National Institute of Child Health and Human Development (NICHD), November 2012. Reviewed March 2017.

What Do We Mean By "Media?"[2]

The term "media" refers to all the many ways people express ideas and convey information. Television, radio, computers, cell phones, newspapers, books, magazines, billboards, music, theater, posters, letters, and the Internet are all examples of media. More recent trends that have transformed the traditional media world include cell phone cameras and mobile texts, social networking and video sharing sites, and blogs and microblogs (blogs with very short posts, like Twitter accounts). These new media share two constants: they are always changing, and they are highly influential, especially in the lives of young people. Recognizing the ever-evolving nature of new media, Media-Smart Youth discusses media forms in general, allowing facilitators and youth to bring in specific types of media relevant to their experiences.

Media And Childhood Obesity

Children today spend as much as four and a half hours each day watching television and are influenced by the programming and advertising they see. In 2010, one out of every three American children is obese or overweight. As childhood obesity rises, there is an opportunity for the Federal communications commission (FCC) to examine the impact of the media and children's television programming on this growing health concern.

Did you know?

- One in every three children (31.7%) ages 2–19 is overweight or obese.
- Obesity is estimated to cause 112,000 deaths per year in the United States.
- One third of all children born in the year 2000 are expected to develop diabetes during their lifetime.
- The effects of childhood obesity create an estimated $3 billion per year in direct medical costs.

Weight Bias And The Media[1]

Children's media have a prevailing tendency to represent positive messages about being thin and negative messages about being overweight. In children's entertainment, thin characters are ascribed desirable attributes and dominate central roles, whereas overweight characters are onscreen rarely or in minor stereotypical roles. Compared with thin characters appearing on television, heavier characters rarely are portrayed in romantic relationships (and never with thin characters), are more likely to be objects of humor and ridicule, and often engage in stereotypical eating behaviors.

Why Do We Need Media-Smart Youth?[2]

Every day, young people actively engage with the media world around them. Today's media world has expanded beyond the traditional forms, such as television, radio, and movies, to include video games, social networking sites, and online videos—all constantly accessible on mobile platforms, such as cell phones. A large-scale national survey found that, in the United States, youth ages 11 to 14 spend an average of 8 hours and 40 minutes each day using media. Through this exposure, young people encounter a barrage of marketing and advertising messages. Depending on their age, children are exposed to between 14,000 and 30,000 ads on TV alone per year. The majority of the advertisements they view are for food, primarily candy, cereal, and fast food.

Importance Of Media Literacy

The influence of the media should not be underestimated. By mid-adolescence, teens have watched many thousands of hours of television—more time than they spend with teachers in school. Add to that figure the hours devoted to surfing the Internet, playing video games, watching videos and DVDs, listening to the radio, and attending movies, and the media's effect becomes clear.

By helping our teens become media literate, we can help protect them from pressures from advertising and other media forms to smoke, drink, use drugs, have sex, or eat unhealthy foods. We also can help them build communication skills, encourage them to consider multiple interpretations of media messages, put portrayals of themselves and others in perspective, and improve media use habits, such as changing ritualistic viewing behaviors. In addition, we can improve the media use habits of the entire family and promote more proactive behavior among all family members.

Media literacy is not media bashing; the goal is not to ridicule the media. Media are dominant forces in our culture and an important part of our teenagers' lives. Media should be evaluated fairly, not denigrated. Media literacy is also no silver bullet or magic wand; it will not instantly solve all of our problems. But it is our best defense in resisting manipulation and keeping a perspective on the images and messages that are a part of media and youth culture.

As you employ these skills at home, remember that the heart of media literacy lies in the discussion. There are many activities that you can do with your children, but nothing is more important than talking with them about what we watch, hear, and read. Keep discussions relaxed; this takes the pressure off of teens to get the "right" answer. Draw out their ideas and guide them to critically examine what they see and hear. Remember to keep probing the answer, as this helps young people expand their thoughts. This helps them focus and helps us understand how they perceive what they view. It doesn't matter so much what questions you ask; the important thing is to get youth to express and challenge what they see and hear.

Young people can learn how to read between the lines so that they can understand exactly what music videos, movies, and other forms of communication that reach youth are saying to them. The media literacy ladder is a good way to organize the discussion.

Rising use of media, which is tied to an increasingly sedentary lifestyle, and exposure to marketing messages for less nutritious food have combined to contribute to rising rates of childhood overweight and obesity. According to a study, about one-third of American children and adolescents ages 2 to 19 are overweight or obese and many more young people are at risk. Too often, children are consuming too many calories while not getting enough of certain nutrients, including calcium, vitamin D, and fiber. Nationwide, fewer than one-third of all children ages 6 to 17 engage in vigorous physical activity.

In response to these trends, several federal agencies have developed programs to help young people make choices that reinforce healthy behaviors, including being physically active and eating nutritious foods. Media-Smart Youth is part of those efforts.

FCC Recommendations

Here are some of the report recommendations on how changes in food marketing can decrease childhood obesity:

- All media and entertainment companies should limit the licensing of their popular characters to food and beverages that are healthy and consistent with nutrition standards.

- The food and entertainment industries should jointly adopt meaningful, uniform nutrition standards for marketing food and beverages to children, as well as a uniform standard for what constitutes marketing to children.

- Industry should provide technology to help consumers distinguish between advertisements for healthy and unhealthy foods and to limit their children's exposure to unhealthy food advertisements.

- If voluntary efforts to limit the marketing of unhealthy foods to children do not help, the FCC should consider revisiting and modernizing rules on commercial time permitted during children's programming.

(Source: "Media And Childhood Obesity," Federal Communications Commission (FCC).)

Chapter 9

Eating Disorders Among Teens: A Cause Of Worry

More than 12 percent of people in the United States—almost 42 million—are between the ages of 10 and 19. These adolescents are increasingly diverse and reflect the changing racial/ethnic, socioeconomic, and geographic structure of the U.S. population.

Number Of Adolescents

Today, adolescents make up 13.2 percent of the population. As the U.S. population ages, adolescents will represent a smaller proportion of the total. By 2050, estimates show that adolescents will make up 11.2 percent of the population. While adolescents are predicted to represent a smaller portion of the total population, estimates show that the number of adolescents in the population will continue to grow, reaching almost 45 million in 2050.

Age And Gender

There are important developmental, physical, and behavioral differences between younger (10–14) and older (15–19) adolescents. For instance, older youth are more likely to engage in unsafe behaviors—including drug use and risky sexual activity—than are younger teens.

There are also differences between male and female adolescents in risky health behaviors. For example, male adolescents are more likely to use tobacco, alcohol, and other drugs while female adolescents are more likely to be physically inactive and to engage in unhealthy eating

About This Chapter: Text in this chapter begins with excerpts from "The Changing Face Of America's Adolescents," U.S. Department of Health and Human Services (HHS), January 4, 2017; Text under the heading "Most Teens With Eating Disorders Go Without Treatment" is excerpted from "Most Teens With Eating Disorders Go Without Treatment," National Institute of Mental Health (NIMH), March 7, 2011. Reviewed March 2017.

behaviors (such as intentionally vomiting and skipping meals), which often leads to eating disorders to control their weight and body composition.

Most Teens With Eating Disorders Go Without Treatment

Results Of The Study

According to the data, 0.3 percent of youth have been affected by anorexia, 0.9 percent by bulimia, and 1.6 percent by binge eating disorder. The researchers also tracked the rate of some forms of eating disorders not otherwise specified (ED-NOS), a catch-all category of symptoms that do not meet full criteria for specific disorders but still impact a person's life. ED-NOS is the most common eating disorder diagnosis. Overall, another 0.8 percent had subthreshold anorexia, and another 2.5 percent had symptoms of subthreshold binge eating disorder.

In addition,

- Hispanics reported the highest rates of bulimia, while Whites reported the highest rates of anorexia.

- The majority who had an eating disorder also met criteria for at least one other psychiatric disorder such as depression.

- Each eating disorder was associated with higher levels of suicidal thinking compared to those without an eating disorder.

Significance

The prevalence of these disorders and their association with coexisting disorders, role impairment, and suicidal thinking suggest that eating disorders represent a major public health concern. In addition, the significant rates of subthreshold eating conditions support the notion that eating disorders tend to exist along a spectrum and may be better recognized by doctors if they included a broader range of symptoms. In addition, the findings clearly underscore the need for better access to treatment specifically for eating disorders.

Bullying And Binge Eating Disorder (BED)

Bullying

Bullying is unwanted, aggressive behavior among school aged children that involves a real or perceived power imbalance. The behavior is repeated, or has the potential to be repeated, over time. Both kids who are bullied and who bully others may have serious, lasting problems.

There are three types of bullying:

Verbal bullying is saying or writing mean things. Verbal bullying includes:

- Teasing
- Name-calling
- Inappropriate sexual comments
- Taunting
- Threatening to cause harm

Social bullying, sometimes referred to as relational bullying, involves hurting someone's reputation or relationships. Social bullying includes:

- Leaving someone out on purpose
- Telling other children not to be friends with someone
- Spreading rumors about someone
- Embarrassing someone in public

About This Chapter: Text under the heading "Weight-Based Bullying And Binge Eating Disorder" is excerpted from "Bullying And Binge Eating Disorder (BED)," StopBullying.gov, U.S. Department of Health and Human Services (HHS), May 12, 2015; Text under the heading "Bullying And Body Image" is excerpted from "Bullying And Body Image," StopBullying.gov, U.S. Department of Health and Human Services (HHS), July 1, 2013. Reviewed March 2017.

Physical bullying involves hurting a person's body or possessions.

Physical bullying includes:

- Hitting/kicking/pinching
- Spitting
- Tripping/pushing
- Taking or breaking someone's things
- Making mean or rude hand gestures

(Source: "Bullying Definition," StopBullying.gov, U.S. Department of Health and Human Services (HHS).)

Weight-Based Bullying And Binge Eating Disorder

Bullying has very serious consequences. Studies show bullying of any kind, but particularly weight-based bullying, leads to increased occurrence of low self-esteem, poor body image, social isolation, eating disorders, and poor academic performance.

Kids and teens who are overweight can be victims of many forms of bullying, including physical force, name calling, derogatory comments, being ignored or excluded, or being made fun of.

Based on a research it was found that:

- Weight-based teasing predicted binge eating at five years of follow-up among both men and women, even after controlling for age, race/ethnicity, and socioeconomic status.
- Peer victimization can be directly predicted by weight.
- 64 percent of students enrolled in weight-loss programs reported experiencing weight-based victimization.
- One third of girls and one fourth of boys report weight-based teasing from peers, but prevalence rates increase to approximately 60 percent among the heaviest students.
- 84 percent of students observed students perceived as overweight being called names or getting teased during physical activities.

Bullying Is Trauma And Can Lead To Binge Eating Disorder

Bullying because of body size can have a major negative impact on this vulnerable population. We know BED has the highest rate of trauma of all eating disorders. That is, individuals who have binge eating disorder have experienced trauma at some point during their lives. Types of trauma include emotional, physical, and sexual abuse, a divorce or death, and, yes, bullying.

Trauma doesn't have to be catastrophic to have lasting catastrophic effects on a person's psychological, social, and physical health.

People living in larger bodies experience trauma every day by being assaulted by negative attitudes and messages about weight from all angles: in the media; at home, school, and work; even in doctors' offices. This increases stress and leads to internalized weight stigma, which further entrenches disordered eating patterns.

Bullying And Body Image

Although bullying can occur among individuals of any weight, overweight and under-weight children tend to be at higher risk for bullying. Targets of verbal bullying based on weight, sometimes referred to as "weight teasing," can experience a number of negative consequences, including a change in body perception.

Weight teasing by both family and peers has been associated with high levels of anxiety and low self-esteem among adolescents. Having low self-esteem because of peer criticism can change an individual's body image. Body image is the positive or negative feelings you have about the way you look.

A study in the *Journal of Pediatric Psychology* found that adolescents teased about weight tended to have a body image that was more negative than those not teased because of weight. Victims of weight teasing who have a negative body image may be at a higher risk for developing unhealthy eating and exercising habits. This could lead to disorders such as anorexia, bulimia, or binge eating.

How Can I Encourage A Healthy Body Image Among Adolescents?

- Promote healthy eating and exercise habits.

- Encourage adolescents not to compare themselves to their peers.

- Set a good example by not criticizing your own body or the bodies of others.

- Help victims of bullying boost self-esteem by focusing on their positive attributes.

- Encourage them to do the things they love. This boosts confidence and builds healthy friendships.

Chapter 11
Weight Loss And Nutrition Myths

"Lose 30 pounds in 30 days!"

"Eat as much as you want and still lose weight!"

"Try the thigh buster and lose inches fast!"

Have you heard these claims before? A large number of diets and tools are available, but their quality may vary. It can be hard to know what to believe.

This chapter discusses myths and provide facts and tips about weight loss, nutrition, and physical activity. This information may help you make healthy changes in your daily habits. You can also talk to your healthcare provider. She or he can help you if you have other questions or you want to lose weight. A registered dietitian may also give you advice on a healthy eating plan and safe ways to lose weight and keep it off.

Weight Loss And Diet Myths

Myth: Fad diets will help me lose weight and keep it off.

Fact: Fad diets are not the best way to lose weight and keep it off. These diets often promise quick weight loss if you strictly reduce what you eat or avoid some types of foods. Some of these diets may help you lose weight at first. But these diets are hard to follow. Most people quickly get tired of them and regain any lost weight.

Fad diets may be unhealthy. They may not provide all of the nutrients your body needs. Also, losing more than 3 pounds a week after the first few weeks may increase your chances of

About This Chapter: This chapter includes text excerpted from "Weight-Loss And Nutrition Myths," National Institute of Diabetes and Digestive and Kidney Diseases (NIDDK), October 2014.

developing gallstones (solid matter in the gallbladder that can cause pain). Being on a diet of fewer than 800 calories a day for a long time may lead to serious heart problems.

TIP: Research suggests that safe weight loss involves combining a reduced-calorie diet with physical activity to lose 1/2 to 2 pounds a week (after the first few weeks of weight loss). Make healthy food choices. Eat small portions. Build exercise into your daily life. Combined, these habits may be a healthy way to lose weight and keep it off. These habits may also lower your chances of developing heart disease, high blood pressure, and type 2 diabetes.

Myth: Grain products such as bread, pasta, and rice are fattening. I should avoid them when trying to lose weight.

Fact: A grain product is any food made from wheat, rice, oats, cornmeal, barley, or another cereal grain. Grains are divided into two subgroups, whole grains and refined grains. Whole grains contain the entire grain kernel—the bran, germ, and endosperm. Examples include brown rice and whole-wheat bread, cereal, and pasta. Refined grains have been milled, a process that removes the bran and germ. This is done to give grains a finer texture and improve their shelf life, but it also removes dietary fiber, iron, and many B vitamins.

People who eat whole grains as part of a healthy diet may lower their chances of developing some chronic diseases. Government dietary guidelines advise making half your grains whole grains. For example, choose 100 percent whole-wheat bread instead of white bread, and brown rice instead of white rice.

TIP: To lose weight, reduce the number of calories you take in and increase the amount of physical activity you do each day. Create and follow a healthy eating plan that replaces less healthy options with a mix of fruits, veggies, whole grains, protein foods, and low-fat dairy:

- Eat a mix of fat-free or low-fat milk and milk products, fruits, veggies, and whole grains.
- Limit added sugars, cholesterol, salt (sodium), and saturated fat.
- Eat low-fat protein: beans, eggs, fish, lean meats, nuts, and poultry.

Meal Myths

Myth: Some people can eat whatever they want and still lose weight.

Fact: To lose weight, you need to burn more calories than you eat and drink. Some people may seem to get away with eating any kind of food they want and still lose weight. But those people, like everyone, must use more energy than they take in through food and drink to lose weight.

A number of factors such as your age, genes, medicines, and lifestyle habits may affect your weight. If you would like to lose weight, speak with your healthcare provider about factors that may affect your weight. Together, you may be able to create a plan to help you reach your weight and health goals.

Eat The Rainbow!

When making half of your plate fruits and veggies, choose foods with vibrant colors that are packed with fiber, minerals, and vitamins.

Red: bell peppers, cherries, cranberries, onions, red beets, strawberries, tomatoes, watermelon

Green: avocado, broccoli, cabbage, cucumber, dark lettuce, grapes, honeydew, kale, kiwi, spinach, zucchini

Orange and yellow: apricots, bananas, carrots, mangoes, oranges, peaches, squash, sweet potatoes

Blue and purple: blackberries, blueberries, grapes, plums, purple cabbage, purple carrots, purple potatoes

TIP: When trying to lose weight, you can still eat your favorite foods as part of a healthy eating plan. But you must watch the **total number of calories** that you eat. Reduce your portion sizes. Find ways to limit the calories in your favorite foods. For example, you can bake foods rather than frying them. Use low-fat milk in place of cream. Make half of your plate fruits and veggies.

Myth: "Low-fat" or "fat-free" means no calories.

Fact: A serving of low-fat or fat-free food may be lower in calories than a serving of the full-fat product. But many processed low-fat or fat-free foods have just as many calories as the full-fat versions of the same foods—or even more calories. These foods may contain added flour, salt, starch, or sugar to improve flavor and texture after fat is removed. These items add calories.

TIP: Read the Nutrition Facts label on a food package to find out how many calories are in a serving. Check the serving size, too—it may be less than you are used to eating.

Myth: Fast foods are always an unhealthy choice. You should not eat them when dieting.

Fact: Many fast foods are unhealthy and may affect weight gain. However, if you do eat fast food, choose menu options with care. Both at home and away, choose healthy foods that are nutrient-rich, low in calories, and small in portion size.

What Is The Difference Between A Serving And A Portion?

The U.S. Food and Drug Administration (FDA) Nutrition Facts Label appears on most packaged foods. It tells you how many calories and servings are in a box or can. The serving size varies from product to product.

A portion is how much food you choose to eat at one time, whether in a restaurant, from a package, or at home. Sometimes the serving size and portion size match; sometimes they do not.

You can use the Nutrition Facts Label:

- to track your calorie intake and number of servings
- to make healthy food choices by serving smaller portions and selecting items lower in fats, salt, and sugar and higher in fiber and vitamins

TIP: To choose healthy, low-calorie options, check the nutrition facts. These are often offered on the menu or on restaurant websites. And know that the nutrition facts often do not include sauces and extras. Try these tips:

- Avoid "value" combo meals, which tend to have more calories than you need in one meal.
- Choose fresh fruit items or nonfat yogurt for dessert.
- Limit your use of toppings that are high in fat and calories, such as bacon, cheese, regular mayonnaise, salad dressings, and tartar sauce.
- Pick steamed or baked items over fried ones.
- Sip on water or fat-free milk instead of soda.

Myth: If I skip meals, I can lose weight.

Fact: Skipping meals may make you feel hungrier and lead you to eat more than you normally would at your next meal. In particular, studies show a link between skipping breakfast and obesity. People who skip breakfast tend to be heavier than people who eat a healthy breakfast.

TIP: Choose meals and snacks that include a variety of healthy foods. Try these examples:

- For a quick breakfast, make oatmeal with low-fat milk, topped with fresh berries. Or eat a slice of whole-wheat toast with fruit spread.
- Pack a healthy lunch each night, so you won't be tempted to rush out of the house in the morning without one.

- For healthy nibbles, pack a small low-fat yogurt, a couple of whole-wheat crackers with peanut butter, or veggies with hummus.

Myth: Eating healthy food costs too much.

Fact: Eating better does not have to cost a lot of money. Many people think that fresh foods are healthier than canned or frozen ones. For example, some people think that spinach is better for you raw than frozen or canned. However, canned or frozen fruits and veggies provide as many nutrients as fresh ones, at a lower cost. Healthy options include low-salt canned veggies and fruit canned in its own juice or water-packed. Remember to rinse canned veggies to remove excess salt. Also, some canned seafood, like tuna, is easy to keep on the shelf, healthy, and low-cost. And canned, dried, or frozen beans, lentils, and peas are also healthy sources of protein that are easy on the wallet.

TIP: Check the nutrition facts on canned, dried, and frozen items. Look for items that are high in calcium, fiber, potassium, protein, and vitamin D. Also check for items that are low in added sugars, saturated fat, and sodium.

Food Myths

Myth: Eating meat is bad for my health and makes it harder to lose weight.

Fact: Eating lean meat in small amounts can be part of a healthy plan to lose weight. Chicken, fish, pork, and red meat contain some cholesterol and saturated fat. But they also contain healthy nutrients like iron, protein, and zinc.

TIP: Choose cuts of meat that are lower in fat, and trim off all the fat you can see. Meats that are lower in fat include chicken breast, pork loin and beef round steak, flank steak, and extra lean ground beef. Also, watch portion size. Try to eat meat or poultry in portions of 3 ounces or less. Three ounces is about the size of a deck of cards.

Myth: Dairy products are fattening and unhealthy.

Fact: Fat-free and low-fat cheese, milk, and yogurt are just as healthy as whole-milk dairy products, and they are lower in fat and calories. Dairy products offer protein to build muscles and help organs work well, and calcium to strengthen bones. Most milk and some yogurts have extra vitamin D added to help your body use calcium. Most Americans don't get enough calcium and vitamin D. Dairy is an easy way to get more of these nutrients.

TIP: Based on Government guidelines, you should try to have 3 cups a day of fat-free or low-fat milk or milk products. This can include soy beverages fortified with vitamins. If you can't digest lactose (the sugar found in dairy products), choose lactose-free or low-lactose dairy products or other foods and beverages that have calcium and vitamin D:

- calcium: soy-based beverages or tofu made with calcium sulfate; canned salmon; dark leafy greens like collards or kale

- vitamin D: cereals or soy-based beverages

Myth: "Going vegetarian" will help me lose weight and be healthier.

Fact: Research shows that people who follow a vegetarian eating plan, on average, eat fewer calories and less fat than non-vegetarians. Some research has found that vegetarian-style eating patterns are associated with lower levels of obesity, lower blood pressure, and a reduced risk of heart disease.

Vegetarians also tend to have lower body mass index (BMI) scores than people with other eating plans. (The BMI measures body fat based on a person's height in relation to weight). But vegetarians—like others—can make food choices that impact weight gain, like eating large amounts of foods that are high in fat or calories or low in nutrients.

The types of vegetarian diets eaten in the United States can vary widely. Vegans do not consume any animal products, while lacto-ovo vegetarians eat milk and eggs along with plant foods. Some people have eating patterns that are mainly vegetarian but may include small amounts of meat, poultry, or seafood.

TIP: If you choose to follow a vegetarian eating plan, be sure you get enough of the nutrients that others usually take in from animal products such as cheese, eggs, meat, and milk. Nutrients that may be lacking in a vegetarian diet are listed in the sidebar, along with foods and beverages that may help you meet your body's needs for these nutrients.

Table 11.1. Common Sources Of Nutrients

Nutrient	Common Sources
Calcium	dairy products, soy beverages with added calcium, tofu made with calcium sulfate, collard greens, kale, broccoli
Iron	cashews, spinach, lentils, chickpeas, bread or cereal with added iron
Protein	eggs, dairy products, beans, peas, nuts, seeds, tofu, tempeh, soy-based burgers
Vitamin B12	eggs, dairy products, fortified cereal or soy beverages, tempeh, miso (tempeh and miso are foods made from soybeans)

Table 11.1. Continued

Nutrient	Common Sources
Vitamin D	foods and beverages with added vitamin D, including milk, soy beverages, or cereal
Zinc	whole grains (check the ingredients list on product labels for the words "whole" or "whole grain" before the grain ingredient's name), nuts, tofu, leafy greens (spinach, cabbage, lettuce)

Part Two
Understanding Eating Disorders
And Body Image Disorders

Chapter 12
Anorexia Nervosa

What Is Anorexia Nervosa?

A person with anorexia nervosa, often called anorexia, has an intense fear of gaining weight. Someone with anorexia thinks about food a lot and limits the food she or he eats, even though she or he is too thin. Anorexia is more than just a problem with food. It's a way of using food or starving oneself to feel more in control of life and to ease tension, anger, and anxiety. Most people with anorexia are female. An anorexic:

- Has a low body weight for her or his height

- Resists keeping a normal body weight

- Has an intense fear of gaining weight

- Thinks she or he is fat even when very thin

- Misses 3 menstrual periods in a row (for girls/women who have started having their periods)

Who Becomes Anorexic?

While anorexia mostly affects girls and women (85–95 percent of anorexics are female), it can also affect boys and men. It was once thought that women of color were shielded from eating disorders by their cultures, which tend to be more accepting of different body sizes. It is not known for sure whether African American, Latina, Asian/Pacific Islander, and American

About This Chapter: This chapter includes text excerpted from "Anorexia Nervosa Fact Sheet," Office on Women's Health (OWH), U.S. Department of Health and Human Services (HHS), July 16, 2012. Reviewed March 2017.

Indian and Alaska Native people develop eating disorders because American culture values thin people. People with different cultural backgrounds may develop eating disorders because it's hard to adapt to a new culture (a theory called "culture clash"). The stress of trying to live in two different cultures may cause some minorities to develop their eating disorders.

What Causes Anorexia?

There is no single known cause of anorexia. Eating disorders are real, treatable medical illnesses with causes in both the body and the mind. Some of these things may play a part:

- **Culture.** Women in the U.S. are under constant pressure to fit a certain ideal of beauty. Seeing images of flawless, thin females everywhere makes it hard for women to feel good about their bodies. More and more, women are also feeling pressure to have a perfect body.

- **Families.** If you have a mother or sister with anorexia, you are more likely to develop the disorder. Parents who think looks are important, diet themselves, or criticize their children's bodies are more likely to have a child with anorexia.

- **Life changes or stressful events.** Traumatic events (like rape) as well as stressful things (like starting a new job), can lead to the onset of anorexia.

- **Personality traits.** Someone with anorexia may not like her or himself, hate the way she or he looks, or feel hopeless. She or he often sets hard-to-reach goals for her or himself and tries to be perfect in every way.

- **Biology.** Genes, hormones, and chemicals in the brain may be factors in developing anorexia.

What Are Signs Of Anorexia?

Someone with anorexia may look very thin. She or he may use extreme measures to lose weight by:

- Making her or himself throw up

- Taking pills to urinate or have a bowel movement

- Taking diet pills

- Not eating or eating very little

- Exercising a lot, even in bad weather or when hurt or tired

- Weighing food and counting calories

- Eating very small amounts of only certain foods

- Moving food around the plate instead of eating it

Someone with anorexia may also have a distorted body image, shown by thinking she or he is fat, wearing baggy clothes, weighing her or himself many times a day, and fearing weight gain.

Anorexia can also cause someone to not act like her or himself. She or he may talk about weight and food all the time, not eat in front of others, be moody or sad, or not want to go out with friends. People with anorexia may also have other psychiatric and physical illnesses, including:

- Depression

- Anxiety

- Obsessive behavior

- Substance abuse

- Issues with the heart and/or brain

- Problems with physical development

What Happens To Your Body With Anorexia?

With anorexia, your body doesn't get the energy from foods that it needs, so it slows down. Look at the picture below to find out how anorexia affects your health.

Can Someone With Anorexia Get Better?

Yes. Someone with anorexia can get better. A healthcare team of doctors, nutritionists, and therapists will help the patient get better. They will:

- Help bring the person back to a normal weight

- Treat any psychological issues related to anorexia

- Help the person get rid of any actions or thoughts that cause the eating disorder

These three steps will prevent "relapse" (relapse means to get sick again, after feeling well for a while).

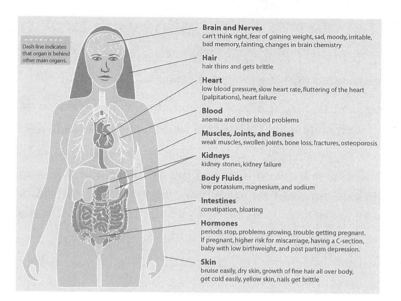

Figure 12.1. How Anorexia Affects Your Whole Body

Some research suggests that the use of medicines—such as antidepressants, antipsychotics, or mood stabilizers—may sometimes work for anorexic patients. It is thought that these medicines help the mood and anxiety symptoms that often co-exist with anorexia. Other recent studies, however, suggest that antidepressants may not stop some patients with anorexia from relapsing. Also, no medicine has shown to work 100 percent of the time during the important first step of restoring a patient to healthy weight. So, it is not clear if and how medications can help anorexic patients get better, but research is still happening.

Some forms of psychotherapy can help make the psychological reasons for anorexia better. Psychotherapy is sometimes known as "talk therapy." It uses different ways of communicating to change a patient's thoughts or behavior. This kind of therapy can be useful for treating eating disorders in young patients who have not had anorexia for a long time.

Individual counseling can help someone with anorexia. If the patient is young, counseling may involve the whole family. Support groups may also be a part of treatment. In support groups, patients, and families meet and share what they've been through.

Some researchers point out that prescribing medicines and using psychotherapy designed just for anorexic patients works better at treating anorexia than just psychotherapy alone. Whether or not a treatment works, though, depends on the person involved and his or her situation. Unfortunately, no one kind of psychotherapy always works for treating adults with anorexia.

What Is Outpatient Care For Anorexia Treatment And How Is It Different From Inpatient Care?

With outpatient care, the patient receives treatment through visits with members of their healthcare team. Often this means going to a doctor's office. Outpatients usually live at home.

Some patients may need "partial hospitalization." This means that the person goes to the hospital during the day for treatment, but sleeps at home at night.

Sometimes, the patient goes to a hospital and stays there for treatment. This is called inpatient care. After leaving the hospital, the patient continues to get help from her healthcare team and becomes an outpatient.

Can Women Who Had Anorexia In The Past Still Get Pregnant?

It depends. When a woman has "active anorexia," meaning she currently has anorexia, she does not get her period and usually does not ovulate. This makes it hard to get pregnant. Women who have recovered from anorexia and are at a healthy weight have a better chance of getting pregnant.

Can Anorexia Hurt A Baby When The Mother Is Pregnant?

Yes. Women who have anorexia while they are pregnant are more likely to lose the baby. If a woman with anorexia doesn't lose the baby, she is more likely to have the baby early, deliver by C-section, deliver a baby with a lower birthweight, and have depression after the baby is born.

What Should I Do If I Think Someone I Know Has Anorexia?

If someone you know is showing signs of anorexia, you may be able to help.

1. **Set a time to talk.** Set aside a time to talk privately with your friend. Make sure you talk in a quiet place where you won't be distracted.

2. **Tell your friend about your concerns.** Be honest. Tell your friend about your worries about her or his not eating or over exercising. Tell your friend you are concerned and that you think these things may be a sign of a problem that needs professional help.

3. **Ask your friend to talk to a professional.** Your friend can talk to a counselor or doctor who knows about eating issues. Offer to help your friend find a counselor or doctor and make an appointment, and offer to go with her or him to the appointment.

4. **Avoid conflicts.** If your friend won't admit that she or he has a problem, don't push. Be sure to tell your friend you are always there to listen if she or he wants to talk.

5. **Don't place shame, blame, or guilt on your friend.** Don't say, "You just need to eat." Instead, say things like, "I'm concerned about you because you won't eat breakfast or lunch." Or, "It makes me afraid to hear you throwing up."

6. **Don't give simple solutions.** Don't say, "If you'd just stop, then things would be fine!"

7. **Let your friend know that you will always be there no matter what.**

Chapter 13
Bulimia Nervosa

What Is Bulimia?

Bulimia nervosa, often called bulimia, is a type of eating disorder. A person with bulimia eats a lot of food in a short amount of time (binging) and then tries to prevent weight gain by getting rid of the food (purging). Purging might be done by:

- Making yourself throw up

- Taking laxatives (pills or liquids that speed up the movement of food through your body and lead to a bowel movement)

A person with bulimia feels he or she cannot control the amount of food eaten. Also, bulimics might exercise a lot, eat very little or not at all, or take pills to pass urine often to prevent weight gain.

Unlike anorexia, people with bulimia can fall within the normal range for their age and weight. But **like** people with anorexia, bulimics:

- Fear gaining weight

- Want desperately to lose weight

- Are very unhappy with their body size and shape

Who Becomes Bulimic?

Many people think that eating disorders affect only young, upper-class white females. It is true that most bulimics are women (around 85–90 percent). But bulimia affects people from all

About This Chapter: This chapter includes text excerpted from "Bulimia Nervosa Fact Sheet," Office on Women's Health (OWH), U.S. Department of Health and Human Services (HHS), July 16, 2012. Reviewed March 2017.

walks of life, including males, women of color, and even older women. It is not known for sure whether African American, Latina, Asian/Pacific Islander, and American Indian and Alaska Native people develop eating disorders because American culture values thin people. People with different cultural backgrounds may develop eating disorders because it's hard to adapt to a new culture (a theory called "culture clash"). The stress of trying to live in two different cultures may cause some minorities to develop their eating disorders.

What Causes Bulimia?

Bulimia is more than just a problem with food. A binge can be triggered by dieting, stress, or uncomfortable emotions, such as anger or sadness. Purging and other actions to prevent weight gain are ways for people with bulimia to feel more in control of their lives and ease stress and anxiety. There is no single known cause of bulimia, but there are some factors that may play a part.

- **Culture.** Women in the United States are under constant pressure to fit a certain ideal of beauty. Seeing images of flawless, thin females everywhere makes it hard for women to feel good about their bodies.

- **Families.** If you have a mother or sister with bulimia, you are more likely to also have bulimia. Parents who think looks are important, diet themselves, or criticize their children's bodies are more likely to have a child with bulimia.

- **Life changes or stressful events.** Traumatic events (like rape), as well as stressful things (like starting a new job), can lead to bulimia.

- **Personality traits.** A person with bulimia may not like herself, hate the way she looks, or feel hopeless. She may be very moody, have problems expressing anger, or have a hard time controlling impulsive behaviors.

- **Biology.** Genes, hormones, and chemicals in the brain may be factors in developing bulimia.

What Are Signs Of Bulimia?

A person with bulimia may be thin, overweight, or have a normal weight. Also, bulimic behavior, such as throwing up, is often done in private because the person with bulimia feels shame or disgust. This makes it hard to know if someone has bulimia. But there are warning signs to look out for. Someone with bulimia may use extreme measures to lose weight by:

- Using diet pills, or taking pills to urinate or have a bowel movement

- Going to the bathroom all the time after eating (to throw up)

- Exercising a lot, even in bad weather or when hurt or tired

Someone with bulimia may show signs of throwing up, such as:

- Swollen cheeks or jaw area

- Calluses or scrapes on the knuckles (if using fingers to induce vomiting)

- Teeth that look clear

- Broken blood vessels in the eyes

People with bulimia often have other mental health conditions, including:

- Depression

- Anxiety

- Substance abuse problems

Someone with bulimia may also have a distorted body image, shown by thinking she or he is fat, hating her or his body, and fearing weight gain.

Bulimia can also cause someone to not act like her or himself. She or he may be moody or sad, or may not want to go out with friends.

What Happens To Someone Who Has Bulimia?

Bulimia can be very harmful to the body. Look at the picture to find out how bulimia affects your health.

Can Someone With Bulimia Get Better?

Yes. Someone with bulimia can get better. A healthcare team of doctors, nutritionists, and therapists will help the patient recover. They will help the person learn healthy eating patterns and cope with their thoughts and feelings. Treatment for bulimia uses a combination of options. Whether or not the treatment works depends on the patient.

To stop a person from binging and purging, a doctor may recommend the patient:

- Receive nutritional advice and psychotherapy, especially cognitive behavioral therapy (CBT)

- Be prescribed medicine

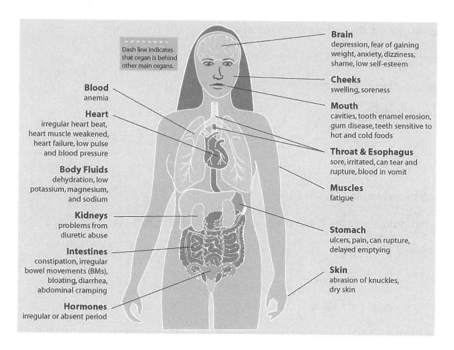

Figure 13.1. How Bulimia Affects Your Body

CBT is a form of psychotherapy that focuses on the important role of thinking in how we feel and what we do. CBT that has been tailored to treat bulimia has shown to be effective in changing binging and purging behavior, and eating attitudes. Therapy for a person with bulimia may be one-on-one with a therapist or group-based.

Some antidepressants, such as fluoxetine (Prozac), which is the only medication approved by the U.S. Food and Drug Administration (FDA) for treating bulimia, may help patients who also have depression and/or anxiety. It also appears to help reduce binge eating and purging behavior, reduces the chance of relapse (to get sick again, after feeling well for a while.), and improves eating attitudes.

Can Women Who Had Bulimia In The Past Still Get Pregnant?

Active bulimia can cause a woman to miss her period sometimes. Or, she may never get her period. If this happens, she usually does not ovulate. This makes it hard to get pregnant. Women who have recovered from bulimia have a better chance of getting pregnant once their monthly cycle is normal.

How Does Bulimia Affect Pregnancy?

If a woman with active bulimia gets pregnant, these problems may result:

- Miscarriage

- High blood pressure in the mother

- Baby isn't born alive

- Baby tries to come out with feet or bottom first

- Birth by C-section

- Baby is born early

- Low birth weight

- Birth defects, such as blindness or mental retardation

- Problems breastfeeding

- Depression in the mother after the baby is born

- Diabetes in the mother during pregnancy

If a woman takes laxatives or diuretics during pregnancy, her baby could be harmed. These things take away nutrients and fluids from a woman before they are able to feed and nourish the baby. It is possible they may lead to birth defects as well, particularly if they are used regularly.

What Should I Do If I Think Someone I Know Has Bulimia?

If someone you know is showing signs of bulimia, you may be able to help.

1. **Set a time to talk.** Set aside a time to talk privately with your friend. Make sure you talk in a quiet place where you won't be distracted.

2. **Tell your friend about your concerns.** Be honest. Tell your friend about your worries about his or her eating or exercising habits. Tell your friend you are concerned and that you think these things may be a sign of a problem that needs professional help.

3. **Ask your friend to talk to a professional.** Your friend can talk to a counselor or doctor who knows about eating issues. Offer to help your friend find a counselor

or doctor and make an appointment, and offer to go with him or her to the appointment.

4. **Avoid conflicts.** If your friend won't admit that he or she has a problem, don't push. Be sure to tell your friend you are always there to listen if he or she wants to talk.

5. **Don't place shame, blame, or guilt on your friend.** Don't say, "You just need to eat." Instead, say things like, "I'm concerned about you because you won't eat breakfast or lunch." Or, "It makes me afraid to hear you throwing up."

6. **Don't give simple solutions.** Don't say, "If you'd just stop, then things would be fine!" Let your friend know that you will always be there no matter what.

Chapter 14
Binge Eating Disorder

Facts On Binge Eating Disorder

Binge eating is when you eat a large amount of food in a short amount of time and feel that you can't control what or how much you are eating. If you binge eat regularly—at least once a week for 3 months, you may have binge eating disorder.

If you have binge eating disorder, you may be very upset by your binge eating. You also may feel ashamed and try to hide your problem. Even your close friends and family members may not know you binge eat.

Binge Eating Disorder Is Different From Bulimia Nervosa

Unlike people with binge eating disorder, people who have bulimia nervosa try to prevent weight gain after binge eating by vomiting, using laxatives or diuretics, fasting, or exercising too much.

How Common Is Binge Eating Disorder?

Binge eating disorder is the most common eating disorder in the United States. About 3.5 percent of adult women and 2 percent of adult men have binge eating disorder. For men, binge eating disorder is most common in midlife, between the ages of 45 to 59.

For women, binge eating disorder most commonly starts in early adulthood, between the ages of 18 and 29. About 1.6 percent of teenagers are affected. A much larger number of adults

About This Chapter: This chapter includes text excerpted from "Binge Eating Disorder," National Institute of Diabetes and Digestive and Kidney Diseases (NIDDK), June 2016.

and children have episodes of binge eating or loss-of-control eating, but the episodes do not occur frequently enough to meet the criteria for binge eating disorder.

Binge eating disorder affects African Americans as often as whites. More research is needed on how often binge eating disorder affects people in other racial and ethnic groups.

Who Is More Likely To Develop Binge Eating Disorder?

Binge eating disorder can occur in people of average body weight but is more common in people with obesity, particularly severe obesity. However, it is important to note that most people with obesity do not have binge eating disorder.

Painful childhood experiences—such as family problems and critical comments about your shape, weight, or eating—also are associated with developing binge eating disorder. Binge eating disorder also runs in families, and there may be a genetic component as well.

What Other Health Problems Can You Have With Binge Eating Disorder?

Binge eating disorder may lead to weight gain and health problems related to obesity. Overweight and obesity are associated with many health problems, including type 2 diabetes, heart disease, and certain types of cancer. People with binge eating disorder may also have mental health problems such as depression or anxiety. Some people with binge eating disorder also have problems with their digestive system, or joint and muscle pain.

What Are The Symptoms Of Binge Eating Disorder?

If you have binge eating disorder, you may:

- eat a large amount of food in a short amount of time; for example, within 2 hours1
- feel you lack control over your eating; for example, you cannot stop eating or control what or how much you are eating

You also may:

- eat more quickly than usual during binge episodes
- eat until you feel uncomfortably full
- eat large amounts of food even when you are not hungry
- eat alone because you are embarrassed about the amount of food you eat
- feel disgusted, depressed, or guilty after overeating

If you think that you or someone close to you may have binge eating disorder, share your concerns with a healthcare provider. He or she can connect you to helpful sources of care.

What Causes Binge Eating Disorder?

No one knows for sure what causes binge eating disorder. Like other eating disorders, binge eating disorder may result from a mix of factors related to your genes, your thoughts and feelings, and social issues. Binge eating disorder has been linked to depression and anxiety.

For some people, dieting in unhealthy ways—such as skipping meals, not eating enough food, or avoiding certain kinds of food—may contribute to binge eating.

How Do Doctors Diagnose Binge Eating Disorder?

Most of us overeat from time to time, and some of us often feel we have eaten more than we should have. Eating a lot of food does not necessarily mean you have binge eating disorder.

To determine if you have binge eating disorder, you may want to talk with a specialist in eating disorders, such as a psychiatrist, psychologist, or other mental health professional. He or she will talk with you about your symptoms and eating patterns. If a healthcare provider determines you have binge eating disorder, he or she can work with you to find the best treatment options.

How Do Doctors Treat Binge Eating Disorder?

Talk to your doctor if you think you have binge eating disorder. Ask him or her to refer you to a mental health professional in your area. A specialist, such as a psychiatrist, psychologist

Is It Safe For Young People To Take Antidepressants For Binge Eating Disorder?

It may be safe for young people to be treated with antidepressants. However, drug companies who make antidepressants are required to post a "black box" warning label on the medication. A "black box" warning is the most serious type of warning on prescription medicines.

It may be possible that antidepressants make children, adolescents, and young adults more likely to think about suicide or commit suicide.

The FDA offers the latest information, including which drugs are included in this warning and danger signs to look for, on their website at www.fda.gov.

(Source: "Binge Eating Disorder Fact Sheet," Office on Women's Health (OWH).)

or other mental health professional, may be able to help you choose the best treatment for you.

Treatment may include therapy to help you change your eating habits, as well as thoughts and feelings that may lead to binge eating and other psychological symptoms. Types of therapy that have been shown to help people with binge eating disorder are called psychotherapies and include cognitive behavioral therapy, interpersonal psychotherapy, and dialectical behavior therapy. Your psychiatrist or other healthcare provider may also prescribe medication to help you with your binge eating, or to treat other medical or mental health problems.

Should You Try To Lose Weight If You Have Binge Eating Disorder?

Losing weight may help prevent or reduce some of the health problems related to carrying excess weight. Binge eating may make it hard to lose weight and keep it off. If you have binge eating disorder and are overweight, a weight-loss program that also offers treatment for eating disorders may help you lose weight. However, some people with binge eating disorder do just as well in a behavioral treatment program designed only for weight loss as people who do not binge eat. Talk with your healthcare professional to help you decide whether you should try to manage your binge eating before entering a weight management program.

A binge eater often:

- Eats 5,000–15,000 calories in one sitting
- Often snacks, in addition to eating three meals a day
- Overeats throughout the day

Chapter 15
Emotional Eating

Emotional eating is a term used to describe the use of food to deal with feelings or, as some experts put it, eating in response to an emotional "trigger." This trigger could be stress, sadness, anxiety, loneliness, anger, or boredom. People who engage in emotional eating often gain weight, because even though food might make them feel better temporarily, the relief doesn't last long, and the underlying emotions remain, compounded by guilt, which causes them to eat more in attempt to feel better again. Surprisingly, emotional eating can even be the result of positive feelings. Many people reward themselves with food after a significant accomplishment or use holidays as an excuse to eat compulsively. Emotional eating is something that most of us do occasionally, such as when cramming for an important test, getting over a breakup, or indulging in a rich dessert on a special occasion, but when it becomes a regular pattern it can be a danger to your health.

Emotional eating and other eating disorders are disturbingly common on college campuses. In a University of Michigan study, 27.8 percent of female undergraduates and 11.8 percent of male undergraduates tested positive for an eating disorder. And yet 82 percent of women and 96 percent of men with eating disorders had not received treatment in the past year.

(Source: "Many Students Diet, Few Seek Treatment for Eating Disorders," University of Michigan, February 4, 2013).

"Emotional Eating," © 2017 Omnigraphics. Reviewed March 2017.

Signs Of Emotional Eating

There are significant differences between emotional eating and eating to satisfy hunger. Some signs of emotional eating include:

- **Suddenness.** Physical hunger tends to come on gradually as the length of time since your last meal increases. But emotional hunger is more sudden, the craving feels urgent, and it's hard to control.

- **Lack of satisfaction.** Normal hunger lessens when you're full, but with emotional eating you tend to eat to the point where you're uncomfortably stuffed.

- **Craving specific foods.** Many types of food can satisfy physical hunger, but emotional eating is characterized by a desire for specific food items, often sweet or fatty things like chips, candy, pizza, or fast-food burgers.

- **Lack of awareness.** Normally, there's a mindfulness to eating. You're aware of the amount of food on your plate, how fast you're eating it, and what's going on around you. With emotional eating, you might be surprised to find that you at an entire bag of chocolate chip cookies without realizing it.

- **Guilt.** When eating to satisfy hunger, you don't have any particular bad feelings about the meal. But emotional eating—especially binging on junk food—can lead to feelings of guilt, regret, or shame.

> A number of experts recommend the "broccoli test" to determine if you're really hungry or emotionally hungry. Ask yourself if you'd eat raw broccoli or some other healthy food, such as fruit. If the answer is yes, then you're actually hungry; if not, then you have an emotional craving.

Causes Of Emotional Eating

There are numerous causes of emotional eating, but some of the most common contributing factors include:

- **Stress.** Stress—especially long-term stress—causes the brain to release a hormone called cortisol, which not only increases appetite, but also can reduce impulse control, making it hard to curb the urge to eat. In addition, studies show that cortisol increases cravings for foods that are high in fat, sugar, or both.

- **Negative emotions.** Many people turn to food as a means of coping with feelings like fear, anger, sadness, anxiety, loneliness, and resentment. The food serves as a distraction and a source of comfort, at least temporarily, allowing them to escape feeling bad for a while.

- **Food as a reward.** Say you've aced a test, so you treat yourself with a chocolate sundae. That's a fairly common way that people reward themselves with food. But there are those who do this habitually, using food as a replacement for other positive experiences that are missing from their lives. Some of these habits go back to childhood, when their parents rewarded them with treats for good behavior.

- **Body image.** People with poor body image often compensate for these feelings by eating. Most often, the negative feelings about their bodies stem from being overweight, so frequent binge eating—especially on junk food—is one of the least healthy ways to overcome these feelings.

- **Social influences.** Cultures all over the world celebrate with food. It's normal to get together with family or friends for a meal and conversation. But some families and some groups of friends tend to put pressure on their members to overindulge on a regular basis. And if one of the members is particularly susceptible to emotional eating, that can create a problem.

Solutions To Emotional Eating

Managing emotional eating means finding healthier ways to process emotions than by indulging in compulsive eating. But that's easier said than done. In practice, controlling ingrained emotional eating habits can be a difficult process, sometimes requiring specialized help. Some ways to break the unhealthy eating cycle include:

- **Relieve stress.** For some people, this can be as simple as calling a friend to chat or playing with a pet, rather than eating during stressful times. Others manage stress through yoga, meditation, music, exercise, massage, or dancing. In some cases, anti-anxiety medication, prescribed by a doctor, may be necessary.

- **Accept emotions.** Bad feelings are part of life, and eating won't change that. Some experts recommend letting yourself experience difficult feelings in order to normalize them. This may not be easy without assistance, so it might be a good idea to work with a therapist, psychologist, or other trained professional.

- **Alternative rewards.** Rather than treating yourself with junk food, find other ways to reward yourself for accomplishments. This might include going to a movie or concert, a weekend trip, a new haircut, new clothes, or a visit to a museum.

- **Be aware.** It's important to be mindful of what you're eating each day. It may be tedious, but one way to do this is to keep a food journal, noting what you ate and why you ate it. Another idea is always to put a controlled amount of food on a plate, and don't go back for seconds. Never eat out of an entire bag of snacks or tub of ice cream. Limiting portions like this can help keep you aware of the amount you're consuming.

- **Don't get overly hungry.** Eat when you're just beginning to get hungry. Being overly hungry is a common way of triggering emotional eating. The best advice is to eat a number of small meals per day, rather than one or two large ones.

- **Get help.** There are therapists who specialize in working with people with eating disorders. They can help you rethink your approach to food, assist with body-image issues, and suggest strategies for coping with emotions. In addition, there are likely a number of support groups in your area where you can get advice and a sympathetic ear as you cope with emotional eating.

> A good first step in controlling emotional eating is to speak with your doctor. He or she may run some simple tests, have useful advice, and can put you in touch with other professionals who can help.

References

1. "Emotional Eating," Waldencenter.org, 2015.

2. "Emotional Eating vs. Mindful Eating: How to Stop Stress Eating and Satisfy Your Needs with Mindfulness," Helpguide.org, February, 2016.

3. Gavin, Mary L., MD. "Emotional Eating," The Nemours Foundation/KidsHealth®, September, 2014.

4. Goldberg, Joseph, MD. "How to Stop Emotional Eating," WebMD.com, May 19, 2016.

5. Kromberg, Jennifer, PsyD. "Emotional Eating? 5 Reasons You Can't Stop," *Psychology Today*, September 18, 2013.

6. Nguyen-Rodriguez, Selena T., PhD, MPH. "Psychological Determinants of Emotional Eating in Adolescence," *Journal of Treatment & Prevention*, April 23, 2009.

7. "Why Stress Causes People to Overeat," *Harvard Mental Health Letter*, February, 2012.

Chapter 16
Night Eating And Sleep Eating Syndromes

Eating disorders do not typically follow clear daily, time-related cycles; however, there are several recognized disorders that involve unusual patterns of eating exclusively during the evening and night hours. Recognizing their unique characteristics may improve diagnosis and treatment.

Night Eating Syndrome

Night eating syndrome (NES), which is also sometimes called nocturnal eating syndrome, is a distinct but only recently recognized disorder. It differs from most other eating disorders in that its symptoms specifically relate to times of the day. Unlike binge eating disorder, in which excessive eating can occur at any time of day, people with NES eat abnormally in very specific patterns.

People with NES typically have little or no appetite in the mornings, and generally do not eat breakfast. They will eat significant amounts in the evening—at least 25 percent of their daily calories—after the dinner meal. Commonly, people with NES will awaken from sleep to eat during the night and feel unable to fall asleep again without eating. People with NES are aware of their behavior, and suffer distress or impairment in functioning as a result. Recognition and treatment of NES is important because NES can significantly worsen obesity. Some studies suggest that obese people with NES have greater difficulty losing weight than those without NES. While cause-and-effect has not been firmly worked out, there is evidence that suggests that NES may precede obesity, and may lead to the development of obesity.

"Night Eating Syndrome And Sleep-Related Eating Disorder," © 2017 Omnigraphics. Reviewed March 2017.

The cause of NES is not known. It tends to occur during periods of increased stress, which may indicate relationships to the factors that underlie mood and anxiety disorders. It is believed that abnormalities in the internal timers that govern sleep-wake cycles are involved. Small studies have suggested that people with NES have abnormal levels and release patterns of brain chemicals involved in sleep, appetite, and mood.

NES is estimated to affect about 1.5 percent of the general population, but, it appears to be much more common in certain subgroups. It has been reported that about 5–15 percent of obese patients have NES, and as much as 42 percent of people considered for weight loss surgery. It is strongly associated with other psychiatric disorders, particularly depression and anxiety. NES may also coexist with other eating disorders. In contrast to most other eating disorders, it appears to affect men and women equally.

Several medications have been tried for NES, with varying degrees of success. The best studied therapies have been selective serotonin re-uptake inhibitor (SSRI) antidepressants such as paroxetine and fluvoxamine, which have shown improvement in some trials. Not all studies have seen success, however. For example, a study of another SSRI, escitalopram, showed no significant benefit in NES. An anti-seizure medication, topiramate, has also been reported to be effective in NES.

Data on non-medication therapy are much more limited. There have been individual case reports of success in NES using psychotherapy. There have also been case reports of improvement with bright light therapy. Neither approach has been studied in trials with large numbers of patients, so it is unknown how effective they are, or how they compare with medical therapy.

There is also very limited data suggesting that weight loss surgery may be effective for NES. More studies are required before this can be widely recommended as treatment for NES.

Sleep-Related Eating Disorder

Despite some superficial similarities, sleep-related eating disorder (SRED) is a quite different condition than NES, both in terms of symptom pattern and underlying causes.

By definition, the nocturnal eating in SRED occurs while the person is asleep. In contrast, patients with NED may leave their bed order to eat, but they are fully awake while they consume food.

SRED is considered a parasomnia. Parasomnias are a class of neurologic disorders that occur during sleep and the transition from wakefulness to sleep. Other disorders of this type include sleep walking, sleep talking, and night terrors.

People with SRED will rise from sleep in a semi-conscious state and proceed to eat or drink. Frequently, they will consume large quantities of food and may open packages or cook while asleep. Some people with SRED eat foods during sleep that they would not eat while awake or make very odd food choices. For example, one patient consumed a potato with mayonnaise and Coca-Cola sauce, while another was reported to have drunk vinegar. In some cases, patients may even eat non-food items or poisonous substances.

People with SRED typically have no memory of their eating episodes, and they may only learn of them when they wake in the morning and find themselves uncomfortably full and the kitchen in disarray. Sleep partners and family members will sometimes observe the episodes and make the patient aware of them.

SRED can be a chronic disorder, and can actually lead to significant weight gain in some cases. The disorder does appear to be more common among the obese, although only a small fraction of obese people are affected.

The cause of SRED is unknown, but is presumed to result in a failure of normal brain mechanisms that prevent active movement during sleep. In keeping with this theory, people with SRED are significantly more likely to sleepwalk or have other types of parasomnias.

The ideal treatment for SRED is not clear; however, several medications including topiramate, pramipexole, and clonazepam have been reported to be effective.

Hypnosedative-Induced Complex Behaviors

In recent years, it has been recognized that certain sedatives can cause sleep behaviors that closely resemble SRED. Affected persons may engage in complex sleep behaviors after taking medication for sleep, including preparing meals, cooking, eating, and even driving. While this looks very much like SRED, these medication-induced cases probably represent a different disorder.

It appears that only a very small proportion of people who take sleep medications develop unusual sleep behaviors. Nevertheless, the widespread use of these medications led the U.S. Food and Drug Administration (FDA) to require warning labels regarding these effects on a number of sleep medications.

The largest number of case reports of unusual sleep behavior have involved zolpidem (Ambien). It is unclear whether zolpidem is particularly likely to cause abnormal sleep behaviors or if this is simply due to the drug's popularity and heavy prescribing. Other drugs reported to cause similar behaviors during sleep include zaleplon (Sonata), triazolam (Halcion), temazepam (Restoril), and ramelteon (Rozerem).

It is unknown why certain people develop abnormal sleep behaviors with these medications, when most do not. Data suggest that the abnormal behaviors may relate to high blood levels of the drugs, either due to taking higher than usual doses or taking other medications that may raise levels of the sleep drug.

In contrast to SREM, abnormal behaviors typically stop when the responsible medication is stopped; however, this can be difficult in patients who are highly dependent on sleeping medications.

Chapter 17
Orthorexia

Those who are obsessed with healthy eating may be suffering from orthorexia nervosa, a term which means literally "fixation on righteous eating." Orthorexia starts out as an innocent attempt to eat more healthfully, but the orthorexic becomes fixated on food quality and purity. They become more and more consumed with what and how much to eat, and how to deal with "slip-ups." An iron-clad will is needed to maintain this rigid eating style. Every day is a day to eat right, be "good," rise above others in dietary prowess, and self-punish if temptation wins (usually stricter eating, fasts, and exercise). Self-esteem becomes wrapped up in the purity of their diet and they often feel superior to others, especially in regards to food intake.

Eventually food choices become so restrictive, with both variety and calories, that health suffers—an ironic twist for a person so completely dedicated to healthy eating. Eventually, the obsession with healthy eating can crowd out other activities and interests, impair relationships, and become physically dangerous.

Is Orthorexia An Eating Disorder?

Orthorexia is a term coined by Steven Bratman, MD, to describe his own experience with food and eating. It is not an officially recognized disorder, but is similar to other eating disorders—those with anorexia nervosa or bulimia nervosa obsess about calories and weight while orthorexics obsess about healthy eating (not about being "thin" and losing weight).

"Orthorexia Nervosa," © 2017 Omnigraphics. Reviewed March 2017.

Why Does Someone Get Orthorexia?

Orthorexia appears to be motivated by health, but there are underlying motivations, which can include safety from poor health, compulsion for complete control, escape from fears, wanting to be thin, improving self-esteem, searching for spirituality through food, and using food to create an identity.

Do I Have Orthorexia?

Consider the following questions. The more "yes" responses, the more likely you are dealing with orthorexia:

- Do you wish that occasionally you could just eat and not worry about food quality?

- Do you ever wish you could spend less time on food and more time on living and loving?

- Does it sound beyond your ability to eat a meal prepared with love by someone else—one single meal—and not try to control what is served?

- Are you constantly looking for the ways foods are unhealthy for you?

- Do love, joy, play, and creativity take a backseat to having the perfect diet?

- Do you feel guilt or self-loathing when you stray from your diet?

- Do you feel in control when you eat the correct diet?

- Have you positioned yourself on a nutritional pedestal and wonder how others can possibly eat the food they eat?

So What's The Big Deal?

The diet of the orthorexic can actually be unhealthy, with the nutritional problems dependent on the specific diet the person has imposed upon him or herself. Social problems are more obvious. An orthorexic may be socially isolated, often because they plan their life around food. They may have little room in life for anything other than thinking about and planning food intake. Orthorexics lose the ability to eat intuitively—to know when they are hungry, how much they need, and when they are full. The orthorexic never learns how to eat naturally and is destined to keep "falling off the wagon" and thus feeling shameful, similar to any other diet mentality.

When Orthorexia Becomes All Consuming

Dr. Bratman, who went through orthorexia, states, "I pursued wellness through healthy eating for years, but gradually I began to sense that something was going wrong. The poetry of my life was disappearing. My ability to carry on normal conversations was hindered by intrusive thoughts of food. The need to obtain meals free of meat, fat, and artificial chemicals had put nearly all social forms of eating beyond my reach. I was lonely and obsessed. I found it terribly difficult to free myself. I had been seduced by righteous eating. The problem of my life's meaning had been transferred inexorably to food, and I could not reclaim it" (Source: www. orthorexia.com).

Are You Telling Me It's Unhealthy To Follow A Healthy Diet?

Following a healthy diet does not mean you are orthorexic, and nothing is wrong with eating healthfully. Unless, however,

1. It is taking up an inordinate amount of time and attention in your life;

2. Deviating from that diet is met with guilt and self-loathing; and/or

3. It is used to avoid life issues.

What Is The Treatment For Orthorexia?

Society pushes healthy eating and thinness, so it is easy for many to not realize how problematic this behavior can become. Even more difficult is that the person doing the healthy eating can hide behind the thought that they are simply eating well (and that others do not). Further complicating treatment is the fact that motivation behind orthorexia is multifaceted. First, the orthorexic must admit there is a problem, then identify what caused the obsession. They must also become more flexible and less dogmatic with their eating. There will be deeper emotional issues, and working through them will make the transition to normal eating easier.

While orthorexia is not a condition your doctor will diagnose, recovery can require professional help. A practitioner skilled at treating those with eating disorders is the best choice. This text can be used to help the professional understand more about orthorexia.

Recovery

The recovered orthorexic will still eat healthfully, but there will be a different understanding of what healthy eating is. They will realize that food will not make them a better person and that basing their self-esteem on the quality of their diet is irrational. Their identity will shift from "the person who eats health food" to a broader definition of who they are—a person who loves, who works, who is fun. They will find that while food is important, it is one small aspect of life and, often, there are things that are more important.

References

1. Ekern, Jacquelyn. "Orthorexia, Excessive Exercise, and Nutrition," Eating Disorder Hope, January 31, 2014.

2. Ekern, Jacquelyn and Karges, Crystal. "How to Recognize Orthorexia?" Eating Disorder Hope, May 17, 2014.

Chapter 18
Pica

What's The Problem?

Pica behavior is the craving to eat nonfood items, such as dirt, paint chips, and clay. Some children, especially preschool children, exhibit pica behavior. Pica behavior is most common in 1- and 2-year old children and usually diminishes with age so that elementary-age children seldom exhibit pica behavior. Soil ingestion is the consumption of soil resulting from various behaviors including, but not limited to, mouthing objects or dirty hands, eating dropped food, and intentionally consuming soil. All children (and even adults) ingest small amounts of soil daily from these behaviors. The distinguishing factor for soil-pica is the recurrent ingestion of unusually high amounts of soil either intentionally by eating dirt or unintentionally from excessive mouthing behavior or eating dropped food. While the typical child might ingest 1/8 teaspoon soil daily (or about 100–200 mg), children with soil-pica behavior ingest about a teaspoon or more of soil daily (or about 1,000–5,000 mg or more per day).

Pica and specifically soil-pica is a public health issue that has gotten little attention because people do not realize that it can lead to significant exposure to chemicals. However, soil ingestion has already been shown to be a significant risk factor for increased blood lead levels (BLL) and for exposure to soil-transmitted parasites. Up to 20 percent of preschool children have soil-pica behavior, which parents may not notice since their preschool children may play unattended in the safety of their back yards.

In addition, pica behavior has also been observed in adults, and in particular pregnant women. In many cases of adult pica, the practice has cultural significance or is the result of

About This Chapter: This chapter includes text excerpted from "Pica Behavior And Contaminated Soil," Centers for Disease Control and Prevention (CDC), February 22, 2011. Reviewed March 2017.

craving during pregnancy. In some cases, the craving is due to a nutritional deficiency, such as iron-deficiency anemia.

An example of an element that may be found in soil is arsenic. Inorganic arsenic doesn't degrade and binds to soil particles at the surface. Historically, repeated applications of arsenic-containing pesticides and herbicides may have increased arsenic levels in top soil to very high concentrations and can be a potential problem for children with soil-pica behavior. Pesticides containing arsenic are no longer commercially available. However, in many cases, soils were treated decades ago, yet the arsenic remains at the surface increasing the risk of contact from children's play activities. If soil ingestion is suspected among children, it is important to know (1) the amount of soil ingested, (2) the frequency of ingestion, and (3) the type of material ingested.

Who's At Risk?

Groups at risk of soil-pica behavior include children aged 6 years and younger as well as individuals of any age who are developmentally delayed. Soil-pica behavior is highest in 1-and 2-year-old children and declines as the children grow older.

Can It Be Prevented?

Parents and guardians must be responsible for closely monitoring young children and persons who have developmental delays to ensure that soil is not ingested. Additionally, proper hand-washing techniques must be employed after being outside and before eating to ensure that contaminants and parasites in soil do not pose any further threats through hand-to-mouth contact.

The Bottom Line

Soil-pica is the ingestion of soil which may lead to exposure to chemicals and has been shown to be a risk factor for exposure to lead and soil-transmitted parasites. Up to 20 percent of preschool children have soil-pica behavior, often consuming soil in their own backyards. Pica behavior can pose significant risks and should be minimized so that those at risk are not harmed by contaminants in the ground. Parents should monitor children when they are playing in the yard and should enforce hand-washing after playing outdoors and before eating.

Chapter 19

Rumination Disorder

What Is Rumination Disorder?

Rumination disorder is the backward flow of recently eaten food from the stomach to the mouth. The food is then re-chewed and swallowed or spat out. A non-purposeful contraction of stomach muscles is involved in rumination. It may be initially triggered by a viral illness, emotional distress, or physical injury. In many cases, no underlying trigger is identified. Behavioral therapy is the mainstay of treatment.

What Are The Symptoms Of Rumination Disorder?

Signs and symptoms of rumination disorder includes the backward flow of recently eaten food from the stomach to the mouth. This typically occurs immediately to 15 to 30 minutes after eating. Rumination often occurs without retching or gagging. Rumination may be preceded by a feeling of pressure, the need to belch, nausea, or discomfort. Some people with rumination disorder experience bloating, heartburn, diarrhea, constipation, abdominal pain, headaches, dizziness, or sleeping difficulties. Complications of severe disorder include weight loss, malnutrition, and electrolyte imbalance.

How Is Rumination Disorder Diagnosed?

Diagnosis can be made by a clinical evaluation of the person's signs and symptoms and history. The following diagnostic criteria is used to aid in diagnosis. These criteria must be met for the last 3 months, with symptoms beginning at least 6 months prior to diagnosis:

- Repeated regurgitation and re-chewing or expulsion of food that

About This Chapter: This chapter includes text excerpted from "Rumination Disorder," Genetic and Rare Diseases Information Center (GARD), National Center for Advancing Translational Sciences (NCATS), April 23, 2015.

- Begins soon after eating

- Does not occur during sleep

- Does not respond to standard treatment for gastroesophageal reflux disease (GERD)

- No retching

- Symptoms are not explained by inflammatory, anatomic, metabolic, or neoplastic processes

These criteria help distinguish rumination syndrome from other disorders of the gastrointestinal tract (GI tract), such as gastroparesis and achalasia where vomiting occurs hours after eating, gastroesophageal reflux where symptoms occur at night, and cyclic vomiting syndrome where the symptoms are chronic/persistent.

Antroduodenal manometry can assist in making and confirming the diagnosis. Antroduodenal manometry involves putting a catheter through the nose into the stomach and small bowel to measure pressure changes.

What Treatments Are Available For Rumination Disorder?

The mainstay treatment of rumination disorder is behavioral therapy. This may involve habitat reversal strategies, relaxation, diaphragmatic breathing, and biofeedback. These types of therapies can often be administered by a gastroenterologist. Other professionals, such as nurse practitioners, psychologists, massage therapists, and recreational therapists may also be involved in care. Ensuring adequate nutrition is essential and treatment will also involve managing other symptoms, such as anxiety, nausea and stomach discomfort (which may involve anti-depressive agents or selective serotonin re-uptake inhibitors (SSRI).

If behavioral therapy is unsuccessful, treatment with baclofen may be considered. There is limited data regarding optimal treatment of rumination disorder, but success with baclofen has been reported.

Where Can I Find More Help?

Nonprofit support and advocacy groups bring together patients, families, medical professionals, and researchers. These groups often raise awareness, provide support, and develop patient-centered information. Many are the driving force behind research for better treatments and possible cures. They can direct people to research, resources, and services. Many groups also have experts who serve as medical advisors.

Chapter 20
Compulsive Exercise

Maintaining Body Weight

Try to maintain your body weight by balancing what you eat with physical activity. If you are sedentary, try to become more active. If you are already very active, try to continue the same level of activity as you age. More physical activity is better than less, and any is better than none. If your weight is not in the healthy range, try to reduce health risks through better eating and exercise habits. Take steps to keep your weight within the healthy range (neither too high nor too low). Have children's heights and weights checked regularly by a health professional.

(Source: "Balance The Food You Eat With Physical Activity—Maintain Or Improve Your Weight," U.S. Department of Health and Human Services (HHS).)

What Is Compulsive Exercise?

Compulsive exercise (also known as anorexia athletica) is a type of addiction in which a person feels that they must work out frequently, often several times a day, and feels anxious and guilty if they don't work out enough. For those struggling with a compulsive exercise disorder, working out is not a choice. Exercise becomes an obligation, one that takes over the person's life to an extreme degree. Working out becomes the most important priority, often at the expense of other activities. A person with compulsive exercise disorder will strive to work out even with an injury or illness that would normally prevent physical exertion. For this reason, compulsive exercise often creates severe physical and psychological problems.

"Compulsive Exercise," © 2017 Omnigraphics. Reviewed March 2017.

Over-Exercising

Too much of a good thing can be very bad for you. Just like eating disorders, societal pressures to be thin can also push women to exercise too much. Over-exercise is when someone engages in strenuous physical activity to the point that is unsafe and unhealthy. In fact, some studies indicate that young women who are compelled to exercise at excessive levels are at risk for developing eating disorders.

Eating disorders and over-exercising go hand-in-hand—they both can be a result of an unhealthy obsession with your body. The most dangerous aspect of over-exercising is the ease with which it can go unrecognized. The condition can be easily hidden by an emphasis on fitness or a desire to be healthy. Like bulimia and anorexia, in which persons deny themselves adequate nutrition by restrictive eating behaviors, over-exercising is a controlled behavior that denies the body the energy and nutrition needed to maintain a healthy weight.

(Source: "Body Image," Office on Women's Health (OWH), U.S. Department of Health and Human Services (HHS).)

Research has shown that the majority of people with compulsive exercise disorder are female. Many people exercise compulsively in order to feel more in control of their lives, and they define their self-worth through athletic achievements. Some use exercise as a way to try to handle difficult emotions or depression, believing that physical exhaustion will eliminate negative feelings. Others develop compulsive exercise disorder through participation in competitive

If You Need To Lose Weight

You do not need to lose weight if your weight is already within the healthy range in the figure, if you have gained less than 10 pounds since you reached your adult height, and if you are otherwise healthy. If you are overweight and have excess abdominal fat, a weight-related medical problem, or a family history of such problems, you need to lose weight. Healthy diets and exercise can help people maintain a healthy weight, and may also help them lose weight. It is important to recognize that overweight is a chronic condition which can only be controlled with long-term changes. To reduce caloric intake, eat less fat and control portion sizes. If you are not physically active, spend less time in sedentary activities such as watching television, and be more active throughout the day. As people lose weight, the body becomes more efficient at using energy and the rate of weight loss may decrease. Increased physical activity will help you to continue losing weight and to avoid gaining it back.

(Source: "Balance The Food You Eat With Physical Activity—Maintain Or Improve Your Weight, U.S. Department of Health and Human Services (HHS).)

sports. External and internal pressure to succeed or excel in sports can drive an athlete to push workouts too far, too frequently. In these cases, exercise compulsion is driven by the belief that additional workouts will provide the edge needed to win.

Health Effects

Compulsive exercise is dangerous and can result in serious physical and psychological harm.

Stress fractures can develop in weight-bearing areas of the body (such as feet and lower legs) as a result of repetitive, high-impact, weight-bearing activities such as running or jumping. Stress fractures produce pain during exercise and can develop into more serious bone breaks if not allowed to heal properly.

Consider This

People who exercise compulsively often believe they are improving their health, but the negative effects of too much exercise can result in serious complications.

Damage to muscle and connective tissue is one common side effect of compulsive exercise. Fitness experts advocate for periods of rest between workouts to allow the body to heal from minor injuries and muscle strains. Long-term damage can result from insufficient rest time, including loss of muscle mass, particularly for those who also struggle with eating disorders. A malnourished body begins to break down muscle tissue for fuel when calories are not available to burn.

Low heart rate (bradycardia) is a condition that develops from metabolic disruptions due to over-exercising. The body's normal response to rapid weight loss is to slow the metabolism in an effort to burn as few calories as possible. Low heart rate typically results in low body temperature and decreased resting heart rate. Low heart rate can easily be mistaken as a positive result of exercise, but in cases of exercise compulsion, low heart rate can produce serious arrhythmias (irregular heart function) and even sudden death.

Osteoporosis results in bone loss which increases the risk of stress fractures. This is a particularly dangerous risk for those suffering from both compulsive exercise and eating disorders, due to malnutrition from a poor diet.

Amenorrhea is the loss of normal menstruation that often develops during rapid and severe weight loss. Amenorrhea can result in loss of bone density and other serious problems including reproductive issues.

Exercising to the point of exhaustion on a frequent basis overloads the body with adrenaline and cortisol hormones, which in turn compromise the body's natural immune system. This increases the likelihood of illness, fatigue, insomnia or other sleep-related problems, irritability, short attention span, and mood swings.

> **Did You Know?**
> Compulsive exercise can lead to other dangerous conditions such as bulimia, anorexia, obsessive-compulsive disorder, negative thinking, low self-esteem, and social isolation.

Signs And Symptoms

Some of the warning signs of a compulsive exercise disorder include:

- Feeling guilty, anxious, or irritable about missing workouts
- Pushing yourself to exercise even when injured or ill
- Persistent exhaustion and fatigue
- Chronic insomnia or disrupted sleep
- Slower than normal heart rate
- Inability to rest or even to sit still
- Giving up social time with friends in order to work out
- Obsessive focus on the number of calories eaten and burned
- Constantly thinking about working out
- Working out even in bad weather
- Low body weight, being underweight for your height
- Feeling obligated to exercise
- Lack of enjoyment of physical activity
- Making up for eating by exercising more
- Lack of satisfaction from personal achievements, always feeling there is more to do

Treatment

Treatment and recovery from compulsive exercise disorder can take months to years, depending on the individual person and situation. Some common treatment approaches include psychotherapy and medication to help manage compulsive disorders. Cognitive-behavioral therapy can help to identify and correct negative thoughts and attitudes. Therapy can also help provide healthy strategies to address negative emotions, stress, low self-esteem and negative body image. Family therapy can be useful when external pressures to excel may have inadvertently caused a compulsive exercise disorder. Family members may not be aware of overly high expectations and the resulting stress that is placed on a young person. This can be particularly critical for athletes who participate in sports that emphasize being thin, such as ice skating, gymnastics, and dancing. Participating in these sports can create an unhealthy focus on body weight.

References

1. "Compulsive Exercise," The Nemours Foundation/KidsHealth®. October 2013.

2. "Compulsive Exercise: Are You Overdoing It?" WebMD. February 26, 2016.

3. "Exercise Compulsion and Its Dangers," Eating Disorder Hope. October 5, 2012.

Chapter 21
Female Athlete Triad

Do You Exercise A Lot?

Being active is great. In fact, girls should be active at least an hour each day. Sometimes, though, a girl will be very active (such as running every day or playing a competitive sport), but not eat enough to fuel her activity. This can lead to health problems.

The following can happen when girls don't eat enough to fuel their activity:

- A problem called "low energy availability"

- Period (menstrual) problems

- Bone problems

These three sometimes are called the female athlete triad. ("Triad" means a group of three.) They sometimes also are called Athletic Performance and Energy Deficit. (This means you have a "deficit," or lack, of the energy your body needs to stay healthy.)

A Problem Called "Low Energy Availability"

Your body needs healthy food to fuel the things it does, like fight infections, heal wounds, and grow. If you exercise, your body needs extra food for your workout.

"Energy availability" means the fuel from food that is not burned up by exercise and so is available for growing, healing, and more. If you exercise a lot and don't get enough nutrition,

About This Chapter: Text under the heading "Do You Exercise A Lot?" is excerpted from "Do You Exercise A Lot?" GirlsHealth.gov, Office on Women's Health (OWH), March 27, 2015; Text under the heading "Amenorrheic Women And The Female Athlete Triad" is excerpted from "Calcium," National Institutes of Health (NIH), November 17, 2016.

you may have low energy availability. That means your body won't be as healthy and strong as it should be.

Some female athletes diet to lose weight. They may do this to qualify for their sport or because they think losing weight will help them perform better. But eating enough healthy food is key to having the strength you need to succeed. Also, your body needs good nutrition to make hormones that help with things like healthy periods and strong bones.

Sometimes, girls may exercise too much and eat too little because they have an eating disorder. Eating disorders are serious and can even lead to death, but they are treatable.

Period (Menstrual) Problems

If you are very active, or if you just recently started getting your period (menstruating), you may skip a few periods. But if you work out really hard and do not eat enough, you may skip a lot of periods (or not get your periods to begin with) because your body can't make enough of the hormone estrogen.

You may think you wouldn't mind missing your period, but not getting your period should be taken seriously. Not having your period can mean your body is not building enough bone, and the teenage years are the main time for building strong bones.

If you have been getting your period regularly and then miss three periods in a row, see your doctor. Not having your period could be a sign of a serious health problem or of being pregnant. Also see your doctor if you are 15 years old and still have not gotten your period.

Bone Problems

Being physically active helps build strong bones. But you can hurt your bones if you don't eat enough healthy food to fuel all your activity. That's because your body won't be able to make the hormones needed to build strong bones.

One sign that your bones are weak is getting stress fractures, which are tiny cracks in bones. Some places you could get these cracks are your feet, legs, ribs, and spine.

Even if you don't have problems with your bones when you're young, not taking good care of them now can be a problem later in life. Your skeleton is almost completely formed by age 18, so it's important to build strong bones early in life. If you don't, then, later on, you could wind up with osteoporosis, which is a disease that makes it easier for bones to break.

Signs Of Not Eating Enough And Eating Disorders

Sometimes, girls exercise a lot and do not eat enough because they want to lose weight. Sometimes, exercising just lowers a person's appetite. And sometimes limiting food can be a sign that a girl may be developing an eating disorder. Here are some signs that you or a friend may have a problem:

- Worrying about gaining weight if you don't exercise enough

- Trying harder to find time to exercise than to eat

- Chewing gum or drinking water to cope with hunger

- Often wanting to exercise rather than be with friends

- Exercising instead of doing homework or other responsibilities

- Getting very upset if you miss a workout, but not if you miss a meal

- Having people tell you they are worried you are losing too much weight

If you think you or a friend has a problem, talk to a parent, guardian, or trusted adult.

Sometimes girls exercise a lot because they feel pressure to look a certain way. Soccer star Brandi Chastain knows how bad that can feel. It took a while, she says, for her to realize that only she was in charge of how she felt about her body. "Body image is tough, but it is something we have to take charge of," Brandi says. "Because inside, only we know who we are."

Tips To Prevent Female Athlete Triad

Eat when you're hungry and include a variety of nutrient-rich foods such as lean sources of protein—lean fish, poultry, beans, nuts, and low-fat dairy products—along with whole grains, fruits, and vegetables. Skipping meals and snacks or severely restricting your food intake will keep you from getting enough calories and other important nutrients such as protein, vitamins, and minerals.

Eat a recovery snack that consists of carbs and protein after your workout. Carbs are your body's primary fuel source to keep you energized, and you need protein to build and repair your muscles.

Talk to a registered dietitian for an individual nutrition plan. A registered dietitian who specializes in sports nutrition can help you choose the best foods and the right amounts to optimize your performance.

(Source: "Are You At Risk For Female Athlete Triad?" Military Health System (MHS).)

Amenorrheic Women And The Female Athlete Triad

Amenorrhea, the condition in which menstrual periods stop or fail to initiate in women of childbearing age, results from reduced circulating estrogen levels that, in turn, have a negative effect on calcium balance. Amenorrheic women with anorexia nervosa have decreased calcium absorption and higher urinary calcium excretion rates, as well as a lower rate of bone formation than healthy women. The "female athlete triad" refers to the combination of disordered eating, amenorrhea, and osteoporosis. Exercise-induced amenorrhea generally results in decreased bone mass. In female athletes and active women in the military, low bone-mineral density, menstrual irregularities, certain dietary patterns, and a history of prior stress fractures are associated with an increased risk of future stress fractures. Such women should be advised to consume adequate amounts of calcium and vitamin D. Supplements of these nutrients have been shown to reduce the risk of stress fractures in female Navy recruits during basic training.

Part Three
Medical Consequences And
Co-Occurring Concerns

Chapter 22
Health Consequences Of Eating Disorders

Eating disorders are serious, potentially life-threatening conditions that affect a person's emotional and physical health. They are not just a "fad" or a "phase." People do not just "catch" an eating disorder for a period of time. They are real, complex, and devastating conditions that can have serious consequences for health, productivity, and relationships.

People struggling with an eating disorder need to seek professional help. The earlier a person with an eating disorder seeks treatment, the greater the likelihood of physical and emotional recovery.

Health Consequences Of Anorexia Nervosa

In anorexia nervosa's cycle of self-starvation, the body is denied the essential nutrients it needs to function normally. Thus, the body is forced to slow down all of its processes to conserve energy, resulting in serious medical consequences:

- Abnormally slow heart rate and low blood pressure, which mean that the heart muscle is changing. The risk for heart failure rises as the heart rate and blood pressure levels sink lower and lower.

- Reduction of bone density (osteoporosis), which results in dry, brittle bones.

- Muscle loss and weakness.

- Severe dehydration, which can result in kidney failure.

About This Chapter: Text in this chapter is excerpted from "Health Consequences Of Eating Disorders," © 2016 National Eating Disorders Association. For more information, visit www.nationaleatingdisorders.org. Reprinted with permission.

- Fainting, fatigue, and overall weakness.

- Dry hair and skin; hair loss is common.

- Growth of a downy layer of hair called lanugo all over the body, including the face, in an effort to keep the body warm.

Health Consequences Of Bulimia Nervosa

The recurrent binge-and-purge cycles of bulimia can affect the entire digestive system and can lead to electrolyte and chemical imbalances in the body that affect the heart and other major organ functions. Some of the health consequences of bulimia nervosa include:

- Electrolyte imbalances that can lead to irregular heartbeats and possibly heart failure and death. Electrolyte imbalance is caused by dehydration and loss of potassium, sodium and chloride from the body as a result of purging behaviors.

- Potential for gastric rupture during periods of binging.

- Inflammation and possible rupture of the esophagus from frequent vomiting.

- Tooth decay and staining from stomach acids released during frequent vomiting.

- Chronic irregular bowel movements and constipation as a result of laxative abuse.

- Peptic ulcers and pancreatitis.

Health Consequences Of Binge Eating Disorder

Binge eating disorder often results in many of the same health risks associated with clinical obesity. Some of the potential health consequences of binge eating disorder include:

- High blood pressure.

- High cholesterol levels.

- Heart disease as a result of elevated triglyceride levels.

- Type II diabetes mellitus.

- Gallbladder disease.

Chapter 23
Obesity And Its Consequences

Overweight And Obesity

Overweight and obesity are increasingly common conditions in the United States. They are caused by the increase in the size and the amount of fat cells in the body. Doctors measure body mass index (BMI) and waist circumference to screen and diagnose overweight and obesity. Obesity is a serious medical condition that can cause complications such as metabolic syndrome, high blood pressure, atherosclerosis, heart disease, diabetes, high blood cholesterol, cancers and sleep disorders. Treatment depends on the cause and severity of your condition and whether you have complications. Treatments include lifestyle changes, such as heart-healthy eating and increased physical activity, and U.S. Food and Drug Administration (FDA) approved weight-loss medicines. For some people, surgery may be a treatment option.

Causes

Energy imbalances, some genetic or endocrine medical conditions, and certain medicines are known to cause overweight or obesity.

Energy imbalances cause the body to store fat

Energy imbalances can cause overweight and obesity. An energy imbalance means that your energy IN does not equal your energy OUT. This energy is measured in calories. Energy IN is the amount of calories you get from food and drinks. Energy OUT is the amount of calories that your body uses for things such as breathing, digesting, being physically active, and regulating body temperature.

About This Chapter: This chapter includes text excerpted from "Overweight And Obesity," National Heart, Lung, and Blood Institute (NHLBI), February 23, 2017.

Overweight and obesity develop over time when you take in more calories than you use, or when energy IN is more than your energy OUT. This type of energy imbalance causes your body to store fat.

Your body uses certain nutrients such as carbohydrates or sugars, proteins, and fats from the foods you eat to:

- **make energy** for immediate use to power routine daily body functions and physical activity.

- **store energy** for future use by your body. Sugars are stored as glycogen in the liver and muscles. Fats are stored mainly as triglycerides in fat tissue.

The amount of energy that your body gets from the food you eat depends on the type of foods you eat, how the food is prepared, and how long it has been since you last ate.

The body has three types of fat tissue—white, brown, and beige—that it uses to fuel itself, regulate its temperature in response to cold, and store energy for future use. Learn about the role of each fat type in maintaining energy balance in the body.

- **White** fat tissue can be found around the kidneys and under the skin in the buttocks, thighs, and abdomen. This fat type stores energy, makes hormones that control the way the body regulates urges to eat or stop eating, and makes inflammatory substances that can lead to complications.

- **Brown** fat tissue is located in the upper back area of human infants. This fat type releases stored energy as heat energy when a baby is cold. It also can make inflammatory substances. Brown fat can be seen in children and adults.

- **Beige** fat tissue is seen in the neck, shoulders, back, chest and abdomen of adults and resembles brown fat tissue. This fat type, which uses carbohydrates and fats to produce heat, increases when children and adults are exposed to cold.

Medical Conditions

Some genetic syndromes and endocrine disorders can cause overweight or obesity.

Genetic Syndromes

Several genetic syndromes are associated with overweight and obesity, including the following.

- Prader-Willi syndrome

- Bardet-Biedl syndrome

- Alström syndrome

- Cohen syndrome

The study of these genetic syndromes has helped researchers understand obesity.

Endocrine Disorders

Because the endocrine system produces hormones that help maintain energy balances in the body, the following endocrine disorders or tumors affecting the endocrine system can cause overweight and obesity.

- **Hypothyroidism**. People with this condition have low levels of thyroid hormones. These low levels are associated with decreased metabolism and weight gain, even when food intake is reduced. People with hypothyroidism also produce less body heat, have a lower body temperature, and do not efficiently use stored fat for energy.

- **Cushing syndrome**. People with this condition have high levels of glucocorticoids, such as cortisol, in the blood. High cortisol levels make the body feel like it is under chronic stress. As a result, people have an increase in appetite and the body will store more fat. Cushing syndrome may develop after taking certain medicines or because the body naturally makes too much cortisol.

- **Tumors**. Some tumors, such as craneopharingioma, can cause severe obesity because the tumors develop near parts of the brain that control hunger.

Medicines

Medicines such as antipsychotics, antidepressants, antiepileptics, and antihyperglycemics can cause weight gain and lead to overweight and obesity.

Talk to your doctor if you notice weight gain while you are using one of these medicines. Ask if there are other forms of the same medicine or other medicines that can treat your medical condition, but have less of an effect on your weight. Do not stop taking the medicine without talking to your doctor.

Several parts of your body, such as your stomach, intestines, pancreas, and fat tissue, use hormones to control how your brain decides if you are hungry or full. Some of these hormones are insulin, leptin, glucagon-like peptide (GLP-1), peptide YY, and ghrelin.

Risk Factors

There are many risk factors for overweight and obesity. Some risk factors can be changed, such as unhealthy lifestyle habits and environments. Other risk factors, such as age, family history and genetics, race and ethnicity, and sex, cannot be changed. Healthy lifestyle changes can decrease your risk for developing overweight and obesity.

Unhealthy lifestyle habits

Lack of physical activity, unhealthy eating patterns, not enough sleep, and high amounts of stress can increase your risk for overweight and obesity.

Lack of physical activity

Lack of physical activity due to high amounts of TV, computer, videogame or other screen usage has been associated with a high body mass index. Healthy lifestyle changes, such as being physically active and reducing screen time, can help you aim for a healthy weight.

Unhealthy eating behaviors

Some unhealthy eating behaviors can increase your risk for overweight and obesity.

- **Eating more calories than you use.** The amount of calories you need will vary based on your sex, age, and physical activity level. Find out your daily calorie needs or goals with the Body Weight Planner.
- **Eating too much saturated and trans fats**
- **Eating foods high in added sugars**

Not enough sleep

Many studies have seen a high BMI in people who do not get enough sleep. Some studies have seen a relationship between sleep and the way our bodies use nutrients for energy and how lack of sleep can affect hormones that control hunger urges.

High amounts of stress

Acute stress and chronic stress affect the brain and trigger the production of hormones, such as cortisol, that control our energy balances and hunger urges. Acute stress can trigger hormone changes that make you not want to eat. If the stress becomes chronic, hormone changes can make you eat more and store more fat.

Age

Childhood obesity remains a serious problem in the United States, and some populations are more at risk for childhood obesity than others. The risk of unhealthy weight gain increases as you age. Adults who have a healthy BMI often start to gain weight in young adulthood and continue to gain weight until 60 to 65 years old, when they tend to start losing weight.

Unhealthy environments

Many environmental factors can increase your risk for overweight and obesity:

- social factors such as having a low socioeconomic status or an unhealthy social or unsafe environment in the neighborhood

- built environment factors such as easy access to unhealthy fast foods, limited access to recreational facilities or parks, and few safe or easy ways to walk in your neighborhood

- exposure to chemicals known as obesogens that can change hormones and increase fatty tissue in our bodies

Family history and genetics

Genetic studies have found that overweight and obesity can run in families, so it is possible that our genes or DNA can cause these conditions. Research studies have found that certain DNA elements are associated with obesity.

Did you know obesity can change your DNA and the DNA you pass on to your children? Learn more about these DNA changes.

Eating too much or eating too little during your pregnancy can change your baby's DNA and can affect how your child stores and uses fat later in life. Also, studies have shown that obese fathers have DNA changes in their sperm that can be passed on to their children.

Race or ethnicity

Overweight and obesity is highly prevalent in some racial and ethnic minority groups. Rates of obesity in American adults are highest in blacks, followed by Hispanics, then whites. This is true for men or women. While Asian men and women have the lowest rates of unhealthy BMIs, they may have high amounts of unhealthy fat in the abdomen. Samoans may be at risk for overweight and obesity because they may carry a DNA variant that is associated with increased BMI but not with common obesity-related complications.

Sex

In the United States, obesity is more common in black or Hispanic women than in black or Hispanic men. A person's sex may also affect the way the body stores fat. For example, women tend to store less unhealthy fat in the abdomen than men do.

Overweight and obesity is also common in women with polycystic ovary syndrome (PCOS). This is an endocrine condition that causes large ovaries and prevents proper ovulation, which can reduce fertility.

Screening And Prevention

Children and adults should be screened at least annually to see if they have a high or increasing body mass index (BMI), which allows doctors to recommend healthy lifestyle changes to prevent overweight and obesity.

Screening for a high or increasing body mass index (BMI)

To screen for overweight and obesity, doctors measure BMI using calculations that depend on whether you are a child or an adult. After reading the information below, talk to your doctor or your child's doctor to determine if you or your child has a high or increasing BMI.

- **Children:** A healthy weight is usually when your child's BMI is at the 5th percentile up to the 85th percentile, based on growth charts for children who are the same age and sex. To figure out your child's BMI, use the Center for Disease Control and Prevention (CDC) BMI Percentile Calculator for Child and Teen and compare the BMI with the table below.

- **Adults:** A healthy weight for adults is usually when your BMI is 18.5 to less than 25. To figure out your BMI, use the National Heart, Lung, and Blood Institute's online BMI calculator and compare it with the table below. You can also download the BMI calculator app for iPhone and Android.

Weight Category	Body Mass Index	
	Children	Adults
Underweight	Below 5th percentile*	Below 18.5
Healthy weight	5th percentile to less than 85th percentile	18.5 to 24.9
Overweight	85th percentile to less than 95th percentile	25 to 29.9
Obese	95th percentile or above	30 or above

Figure 23.1. BMI Table For Children And Adults.

Body mass index (BMI) is used to determine if you or your child are underweight, healthy, or overweight or obese. Children are underweight if their BMI is below the 5th percentile, healthy weight if their BMI is between the 5th to less than the 85th percentile, overweight if their BMI is the 85th percentile to less than the 95th percentile, and obese if their BMI is the

95th percentile or above. Adults are underweight if their BMI is below 18.5, healthy weight if their BMI is 18.5 to 24.9, overweight if their BMI is 25 to 29.9, and obese if their BMI is 30 or above. *A child's BMI percentile is calculated by comparing your child's BMI to growth charts for children who are the same age and sex as your child.

Healthy lifestyle changes to prevent overweight and obesity

If your BMI indicates you are getting close to being overweight, or if you have certain risk factors, your doctor may recommend you adopt healthy lifestyle changes to prevent you from becoming overweight and obese. Changes include healthy eating, being physically active, aiming for a healthy weight, and getting healthy amounts of sleep.

Signs, Symptoms, And Complications

There are no specific symptoms of overweight and obesity. The signs of overweight and obesity include a high body mass index (BMI) and an unhealthy body fat distribution that can be estimated by measuring your waist circumference. Obesity can cause complications in many parts of your body.

High body mass index (BMI)

A high BMI is the most common sign of overweight and obesity.

Weight Category	Body Mass Index	
	Children	Adults
Underweight	Below 5th percentile*	Below 18.5
Healthy weight	5th percentile to less than 85th percentile	18.5 to 24.9
Overweight	85th percentile to less than 95th percentile	25 to 29.9
Obese	95th percentile or above	30 or above

Figure 23.2. BMI Table For Children And Adults.

Body mass index (BMI) is used to determine if you or your child are underweight, healthy, or overweight or obese. Children are underweight if their BMI is below the 5th percentile, healthy weight if their BMI is between the 5th to less than the 85th percentile, overweight if their BMI is the 85th percentile to less than the 95th percentile, and obese if their BMI is the

95th percentile or above. Adults are underweight if their BMI is below 18.5, healthy weight if their BMI is 18.5 to 24.9, overweight if their BMI is 25 to 29.9, and obese if their BMI is 30 or above.

A child's BMI percentile is calculated by comparing your child's BMI to growth charts for children who are the same age and sex as your child.

Unhealthy body fat distribution

Another sign of overweight and obesity is having an unhealthy body fat distribution. Fatty tissue is found in different parts of your body and has many functions. Having an increased waist circumference suggests that you have increased amounts of fat in your abdomen. An increased waist circumference is a sign of obesity and can increase your risk for obesity-related complications.

Did you know that fatty tissue has different functions depending on its location in your body? Visceral fat is the fatty tissue inside of your abdomen and organs. While we do not know what causes the body to create and store visceral fat, it is known that this type of fat interferes with the body's endocrine and immune systems and promotes chronic inflammation and contributes to obesity-related complications.

Complications

Obesity may cause the following complications:

- **Metabolic Syndrome**

- **Type 2 diabetes**

- **High blood cholesterol and high triglyceride levels in the blood**

- **Diseases of the heart and blood vessels** such as high blood pressure, atherosclerosis, heart attacks and stroke

- **Respiratory problems** such as obstructive sleep apnea, asthma, and obesity hypoventilation syndrome

- **Back pain**

- **Non-alcoholic fatty liver disease (NAFLD)**

- **Osteoarthritis**, a chronic inflammation that damages the cartilage and bone in or around the affected joint. It can cause mild or severe pain and usually affects weight-bearing joints in people who are obese. It is a major cause of knee replacement surgery in patients who are obese for a long time.

- **Urinary incontinence**, the unintentional leakage of urine. Chronic obesity can weaken pelvic muscles, making it harder to maintain bladder control. While it can happen to both sexes, it usually affects women as they age.

- **Gallbladder disease**

- **Emotional health** issues such as low self-esteem or depression. This may commonly occur in children.

- **Cancers** of the esophagus, pancreas, colon, rectum, kidney, endometrium, ovaries, gallbladder, breast, or liver.

Chapter 24
Oral Health Consequences Of Eating Disorders

Dental Complications Of Eating Disorders

Dietary habits can and do play a role in oral health. Everyone has heard from their dentist that eating too much sugar can lead to cavities, but did you know that high intake of acidic "diet" foods can have an equally devastating effect on your teeth? Changes in the mouth are oftentimes the first physical signs of an eating disorder. The harmful habits and nutritional deficiencies that often accompany disordered eating can have severe consequences on one's dental health.

An eating disorder may cause lingering or even permanent damage to the teeth and mouth. Early detection of eating disorders may ensure a smoother and more successful recovery period for the body and the teeth. Damage to the teeth and mouth can be tempered by arming yourself with the right information and receiving appropriate guidance from your oral health professional.

If you or your loved one has struggled with an eating disorder, make sure you ask questions about your dental provider's qualifications, their experience, the kinds of cases they have treated and their treatment philosophies. It is important that like all of your relationships with healthcare providers, your relationship with your oral healthcare provider be candid and honest. They can only provide as much help as you allow them to provide.

If you are experiencing any dental symptoms, talk with your dentist about ways to care for your teeth and mouth. If you notice these symptoms in a loved one, you may use your

About This Chapter: Text in this chapter is excerpted from "Dental Complications Of Eating Disorders," © 2016 National Eating Disorders Association. For more information, visit www.nationaleatingdisorders.org. Reprinted with permission.

observations to initiate a respectful conversation about your concerns. There are methods for improving oral health while seeking help to change harmful eating habits.

Dental Effects Of Eating Disorders

- Without the proper nutrition, gums and other soft tissue inside your mouth may bleed easily. The glands that produce saliva may swell. Individuals may experience chronic dry mouth.

- Food restriction often leads to nutritional deficiency. Nutrients that promote oral health include calcium, iron and B vitamins. Insufficient calcium promotes tooth decay and gum disease; even if an anorexia patient does consume enough calcium, they also need enough vitamin D to help the body absorb it. Insufficient iron can foster the development of sores inside the mouth. Insufficient amounts of vitamin B3 (also known as niacin) can contribute to bad breath and the development of canker sores. Gums can become red and swollen—almost glossy-looking—which is often a sign of gingivitis. The mouth can also be extremely dry, due to dehydration, and lips may become reddened, dry and cracked.

- Frequent vomiting leads to strong stomach acid repeatedly flowing over the teeth. The tooth's outer covering (enamel) can be lost and teeth can change in color, shape and length, becoming brittle, translucent and weak. Eating hot or cold food or drink may become uncomfortable. Tissue loss and erosive lesions on the surface of the mouth may occur. The edges of teeth often become thin and break off easily. In extreme cases the pulp can be exposed and cause infection, discoloration or even pulp death. Tooth decay can actually be aggravated by extensive tooth brushing or rinsing following vomiting.

- Degenerative arthritis within the temporomandibular joint in the jaw is a dental complication often associated with eating disorders. This joint is found where the lower jaw hinges to the skull. When arthritis begins in this joint it may create pain in the joint area, chronic headaches and problems chewing and opening/closing the mouth.

- Purging can lead to redness, scratches and cuts inside the mouth, especially on the upper surface commonly referred to as the 'soft palate.' Such damage is a warning sign for dental professionals, because healthy daily behaviors rarely cause harm to this area. Soft palate damage is often accompanied by cuts or bruises on the knuckles as a result of an individual's teeth placing pressure on the skin while attempting to purge.

- A frequent binge-and-purge cycle can cause an enlargement of the salivary glands. Enlarged glands can be painful and are often visible to others, which can lead to emotional distress.

Treatment Of The Oral Health Consequences Of Eating Disorders

- Maintain meticulous oral healthcare related to tooth brushing and flossing, as well as frequent and appropriate communication and examination by your dentist. A confidential relationship should always be maintained between the dentist and patient, and therefore, the patient should feel that the dental office is a "safe" place to disclose their ED struggles and progress towards recovery.

- Individuals in treatment may still engage in purging behaviors, and should be honest with their treatment team about these behaviors. To maintain oral care while curbing these behaviors, after purging patients should immediately rinse their mouth with water or use a sugar-free mouth rinse. Patients should swish only water around their mouth due to the high acidic content in the oral cavity. It has also been recommended that brushing be halted for an hour to avoid actually scrubbing the stomach acids deeper into the tooth enamel.

- A dry mouth, or xerostomia, may result from vomiting and/or poor overall nutrition. Xerostomia will also frequently lead to tooth decay. Moisturizing the mouth with water, or other specified products, will help keep recurrent decay at a minimum.

- Consult with your dentist about your specific treatment needs. Fluoride rinses may be prescribed as well as desensitizing or re-mineralizing agents.

Chapter 25

The Link Between Osteoporosis And Anorexia

What Is Osteoporosis?

Osteoporosis is a condition in which the bones become less dense and more likely to fracture. Fractures from osteoporosis can result in significant pain and disability. In the United States, more than 53 million people either already have osteoporosis or are at high risk due to low bone mass.

Risk factors for developing osteoporosis include:

- thinness or small frame

- family history of the disease

- being postmenopausal and particularly having had early menopause

- abnormal absence of menstrual periods (amenorrhea)

- prolonged use of certain medications, such as those used to treat lupus, asthma, thyroid deficiencies, and seizures

- low calcium intake

- lack of physical activity

- smoking

- excessive alcohol intake.

About This Chapter: This chapter includes text excerpted from "What People With Anorexia Nervosa Need To Know About Osteoporosis," National Institute of Arthritis and Musculoskeletal and Skin Diseases (NIAMS), April 2016.

Osteoporosis often can be prevented. It is known as a silent disease because, if undetected, bone loss can progress for many years without symptoms until a fracture occurs. Osteoporosis has been called a childhood disease with old age consequences because building healthy bones in youth helps prevent osteoporosis and fractures later in life. However, it is never too late to adopt new habits for healthy bones.

What Is Anorexia Nervosa?

Anorexia nervosa is an eating disorder characterized by an irrational fear of weight gain. People with anorexia nervosa believe that they are overweight even when they are extremely thin.

Individuals with anorexia become obsessed with food and severely restrict their dietary intake. The disease is associated with several health problems and, in rare cases, even death. The disorder may begin as early as the onset of puberty. The first menstrual period is typically delayed in girls who have anorexia when they reach puberty. For girls who have already reached puberty when they develop anorexia, menstrual periods are often infrequent or absent.

The Link Between Anorexia Nervosa And Osteoporosis

Anorexia nervosa has significant physical consequences. Affected individuals can experience nutritional and hormonal problems that negatively impact bone density. Low body weight in females can cause the body to stop producing estrogen, resulting in a condition known as amenorrhea, or absent menstrual periods. Low estrogen levels contribute to significant losses in bone density.

In addition, individuals with anorexia often produce excessive amounts of the adrenal hormone cortisol, which is known to trigger bone loss. Other problems, such as a decrease in the production of growth hormone and other growth factors, low body weight (apart from the estrogen loss it causes), calcium deficiency, and malnutrition, may contribute to bone loss in girls and women with anorexia. Weight loss, restricted dietary intake, and testosterone deficiency may be responsible for the low bone density found in males with the disorder.

Studies suggest that low bone mass is common in people with anorexia and that it occurs early in the course of the disease. Girls with anorexia may be less likely to reach their peak bone density and therefore may be at increased risk for osteoporosis and fracture throughout life.

Osteoporosis Management Strategies

Up to one-third of peak bone density is achieved during puberty. Anorexia is often identified during mid to late adolescence, a critical period for bone development. The longer the duration of the disorder, the greater the bone loss and the less likely it is that bone mineral density will ever return to normal. The primary goal of medical therapy for individuals with anorexia is weight gain and, in females, the return of normal menstrual periods. However, attention to other aspects of bone health is also important.

Nutrition. A well-balanced diet rich in calcium and vitamin D is important for healthy bones. Good sources of calcium include low-fat dairy products; dark green, leafy vegetables; and calcium-fortified foods and beverages. Supplements can help ensure that people get adequate amounts of calcium each day, especially in people with a proven milk allergy. The Institute of Medicine recommends a daily calcium intake of 1,000 mg for men and women up to age 50. Women over age 50 and men over age 70 should increase their intake to 1,200 mg daily.

Vitamin D plays an important role in calcium absorption and bone health. Food sources of vitamin D include egg yolks, saltwater fish, and liver. Many people may need vitamin D supplements to achieve the recommended intake of 600 to 800 International Units (IU) each day.

Exercise. Like muscle, bone is living tissue that responds to exercise by becoming stronger. The best activity for your bones is weight-bearing exercise that forces you to work against gravity. Some examples include walking, climbing stairs, lifting weights, and dancing.

Although walking and other types of regular exercise can help prevent bone loss and provide many other health benefits, these potential benefits need to be weighed against the risk of fractures, delayed weight gain, and exercise-induced amenorrhea in people with anorexia and those recovering from the disorder.

Healthy lifestyle. Smoking is bad for bones as well as the heart and lungs. In addition, smokers may absorb less calcium from their diets. Alcohol also can have a negative effect on bone health. Those who drink heavily are more prone to bone loss and fracture, because of both poor nutrition and increased risk of falling.

Bone density test. A bone mineral density (BMD) test measures bone density in various parts of the body. This safe and painless test can detect osteoporosis before a fracture occurs and can predict one's chances of fracturing in the future. The BMD test can help determine whether medication should be considered.

Medication. There is no cure for osteoporosis. However, medications are available to prevent and treat the disease in postmenopausal women, men, and both women and men taking glucocorticoid medication.

Chapter 26

Eating Disorders And Pregnancy

Eating During Pregnancy

Eating healthy foods is more important now than ever! You need more protein, iron, calcium, and folic acid than you did before pregnancy. You also need more calories. But "eating for two" doesn't mean eating twice as much. Rather, it means that the foods you eat are the main source of nutrients for your baby. Sensible, balanced meals combined with regular physical fitness is still the best recipe for good health during your pregnancy.

Foods Good For Mom And Baby

A pregnant woman needs more of many important vitamins, minerals, and nutrients than she did before pregnancy. Making healthy food choices every day will help you give your baby what he or she needs to develop. ChooseMyPlate for pregnant and breastfeeding women can show you what to eat as well as how much you need to eat from each food group based on your height, weight, and activity level.

Talk to your doctor if you have special diet needs for these reasons:

- Diabetes—Make sure you review your meal plan and insulin needs with your doctor. High blood glucose levels can be harmful to your baby.

- Lactose intolerance—Find out about low-lactose or reduced-lactose products and calcium supplements to ensure you are getting the calcium you need.

About This Chapter: Text under the heading "Eating During Pregnancy" is excerpted from "Staying Healthy And Safe," Office on Women's Health (OWH), U.S. Department of Health and Human Services (HHS), February 1, 2017; Text under the heading "Pregnancy And Eating Disorders" is © 2017 Omnigraphics. Reviewed March 2017.

- Vegetarian—Ensure that you are eating enough protein, iron, vitamin B12, and vitamin D.

- PKU—Keep good control of phenylalanine levels in your diet.

Cravings

Many women have strong desires for specific foods during pregnancy. The desire for "pickles and ice cream" and other cravings might be caused by changes in nutritional needs during pregnancy. The fetus needs nourishment. And a woman's body absorbs and processes nutrients differently while pregnant. These changes help ensure normal development of the baby and fill the demands of breastfeeding once the baby is born.

Some women crave nonfood items such as clay, ice, laundry starch, or cornstarch. A desire to eat nonfood items is called pica. Eating nonfood items can be harmful to your pregnancy. Talk to your doctor if you have these urges.

Pregnancy And Eating Disorders

Adequate nutrition is vital during pregnancy to ensure the health and well-being of both mother and baby. As a result, pregnancy may present challenges for women who are struggling with or recovering from eating disorders. Pregnancy creates physical and emotional changes that can be stressful for anyone, but especially for women who have preexisting mental health conditions. Even women who believe they have put their disordered eating behaviors in the past may be vulnerable to relapse due to the bodily changes associated with pregnancy. The normal weight gain during pregnancy can trigger symptoms of anorexia, for instance, while the feelings of fullness as the baby grows can create an urge to purge among people with bulimia. The food cravings that often occur during pregnancy can also be problematic for people with binge eating disorder.

If left untreated during pregnancy, active eating disorders can cause serious complications that jeopardize the health of both mother and baby. Mothers with eating disorders are more likely to deliver by Cesarean section and experience postpartum depression. Meanwhile, babies born to mothers with eating disorders have a high risk of premature delivery, low birth weight, and small head circumference. On the other hand, some women find it easier to avoid disordered eating behavior during pregnancy as their focus shifts to protecting the health and welfare of the fetus. Given the importance of nutrition throughout pregnancy, however, women with eating disorders should seek professional advice and treatment to ensure that the condition does not interfere with the normal growth and development of the baby.

Recognizing The Signs Of Eating Disorders

Eating disorders may impact a woman's reproductive health even before she becomes pregnant. Women with anorexia or bulimia often experience irregularity or cessation of menstrual cycles, for instance, which can affect fertility and reduce the likelihood of conception. Therefore, doctors recommend that women bring eating disorders under control and maintain a healthy weight for several months before trying to get pregnant. Even in such cases, however, some women find that the bodily changes associated with pregnancy may trigger or exacerbate the symptoms of eating disorders. Some of the common signs that a woman is struggling with an eating disorder during pregnancy include:

- weight loss or very limited weight gain throughout the pregnancy
- anxiety about being overweight
- restricting food intake, skipping meals, or eliminating major food groups
- vomiting or purging to get rid of calories consumed
- extreme (to the point of exhaustion) or excessive exercising to stay thin
- chronic fatigue, dizziness, or fainting
- depression, lack of interest in socializing, or avoidance of family and friends

If these signs appear during pregnancy, it is important to seek treatment to ensure a healthy outcome for both mother and baby.

Understanding The Risks Of Eating Disorders

Left untreated, eating disorders can have debilitating effects on the health of both the pregnant woman and the unborn baby. Understanding the risks posed by eating disorders may encourage expectant mothers to get the help they need to have a healthy pregnancy. Some of the potential health risks for a pregnant woman with an eating disorder include:

- severe dehydration or malnutrition
- high blood pressure (preeclampsia), gestational diabetes, or anemia
- cardiac irregularities
- miscarriage, stillbirth, or premature labor
- complications during delivery and increased risk of Cesarean section
- extended time required to heal from childbirth

- postpartum depression

- difficulties breastfeeding

- low self-esteem and poor body image

- social withdrawal, isolation, and marital or family conflicts

Eating disorders also carry a number of serious risks for the developing baby, including:

- malnutrition, abnormal fetal growth, or poor development

- premature birth

- respiratory distress

- small head circumference

- low birth weight (with anorexia or bulimia)

- high birth weight (with binge eating disorder)

- feeding difficulties

The seriousness of these risks, along with the natural maternal instinct to protect the developing baby, enables some women to effectively manage their eating disorders during pregnancy.

Managing Eating Disorders In Pregnancy

For some women, on the other hand, the physical and emotional changes that occur during pregnancy may trigger or worsen eating disorder symptoms. Those with anorexia, for instance, may struggle with their inability to fully control their eating and weight gain while pregnant.

Pregnant women who are struggling with eating disorders should see a counselor or therapist to help guide them through pregnancy-related changes, fears about weight gain, and concerns about body image. In addition, they should work with a nutritionist or dietitian to learn about nutritional requirements during pregnancy, ensure that caloric intake is sufficient to support fetal development, and create appropriate meal plans. Finally, they should inform their obstetrician about their eating disorder and make regular visits to track prenatal growth. The pregnancy may be classified as "high risk" so that the healthcare provider can carefully monitor the health of both mother and baby. Additional tips to help alleviate concerns and manage eating disorders during pregnancy include:

- remember that the source of weight gain is a growing baby

- avoid the scale, and ask the healthcare provider not to share your weight during checkups

- try to ignore, or at least not dwell on, comments others make about your pregnant body

- avoid looking at magazines that feature unrealistic postnatal weight-loss stories

Maintaining Health After Childbirth

Even when women with eating disorders manage to keep them under control during pregnancy, many tend to suffer relapses following childbirth. Women face extreme social pressure to lose pregnancy weight as quickly as possible. As a result, many women feel that they must begin a weight-loss diet or exercise regimen immediately after their baby has been born. This pressure to shed pounds can trigger disordered eating behaviors. Experts recommend focusing instead on the remarkable physical accomplishment of growing and delivering a healthy baby. This focus can help women accept the changes in body shape and appearance that may have resulted from pregnancy and childbirth.

Experts also stress that it is important for women to take care of their own health following childbirth. Women with eating disorders are particularly susceptible to postnatal depression, so they should watch out for symptoms and seek professional help if they appear. Many women with eating disorders also express concerns about their ability to breastfeed. As long as the eating disorder is under control, it should not affect breastfeeding. But it is important to remember that restricting caloric intake during breastfeeding can reduce both the quantity and quality of breastmilk. Adequate nutrition is also important to ensure that new mothers have the energy, health, and well-being necessary to love, care for, and enjoy their infant.

References

1. "Eating Disorders and Pregnancy." Eating Disorder Hope, May 25, 2013.

2. "Eating Disorders and Pregnancy." Eating Disorders Victoria, June 24, 2015.

3. "Pregnancy and Eating Disorders." American Pregnancy Association, July 2015.

Chapter 27
What Is Diabulimia?

Most people are familiar with the more widely known eating disorders anorexia nervosa, bulimia nervosa and even binge eating disorder, but few recognize the link between type 1 diabetes and eating disorders. The term "diabulimia" (also known as ED-DMT1) has often been used to refer to this life-threatening combination and the unhealthy practice of withholding insulin to manipulate or lose weight. People suffering from ED-DMT1 may exhibit any number of eating disorder behaviors or they may only manipulate their insulin and otherwise have normal eating patterns.

This risky practice can have catastrophic health consequences. Often these individuals take just enough insulin to function and consistently feel dehydrated, fatigued and irritable. More critically, they face long-term health complications ranging from blindness and nerve disorders to kidney failure and diabetic ketoacidosis (an acidic buildup in the blood resulting from inadequate insulin levels). ED-DMT1 is a relatively new term and the link between type 1 diabetes and eating disorders is not yet recognized as a medical or psychiatric condition. As a result, it is greatly under-diagnosed and left untreated. The first step in treating this dangerous disorder is understanding the causes and symptoms.

Numerous studies conclude that woman with type 1 diabetes are twice as likely to be diagnosed with an eating disorder compared to their non-diabetic peers. Although many of these studies suggest that there is a higher rate of woman engaging in this risky practice, type 1 diabetic men can and do suffer from eating disorders as well.

There are many factors that can contribute to the increased risk of ED-DMT1: the necessary emphasis on food and dietary restraint associated with the management of type 1 diabetes

About This Chapter: Text in this chapter is excerpted from "What Is Diabulimia?" © 2011-2016 We Are Diabetes. Reprinted with permission.

can create an unhealthy focus on food, numbers, and control. The psychological and emotional effects of having to manage a chronic medical condition such as type 1 diabetes, can also play a role. Depression, anxiety and poor body image are common with the dual diagnosis of ED-DMT1. Living with type 1 diabetes is not easy; sometimes insulin omission or other behaviors that could be considered traits of an eating disorder may start out as an act of diabetes rebellion but can manifest over time into an overwhelming cycle of eating disordered thoughts and symptoms.

Chapter 28
Eating Disorders And Diabetes

What Is Diabetes

Diabetes is a disease that occurs when your blood glucose, also called blood sugar, is too high. Blood glucose is your main source of energy and comes from the food you eat. Insulin, a hormone made by the pancreas, helps glucose from food get into your cells to be used for energy. Sometimes your body doesn't make enough—or any—insulin or doesn't use insulin well. Glucose then stays in your blood and doesn't reach your cells.

Over time, having too much glucose in your blood can cause health problems. Although diabetes has no cure, you can take steps to manage your diabetes and stay healthy.

Sometimes people call diabetes "a touch of sugar" or "borderline diabetes." These terms suggest that someone doesn't really have diabetes or has a less serious case, but every case of diabetes is serious.

Types Of Diabetes

The most common types of diabetes are type 1, type 2, and gestational diabetes.

Type 1 Diabetes

If you have type 1 diabetes, your body does not make insulin. Your immune system attacks and destroys the cells in your pancreas that make insulin. Type 1 diabetes is usually diagnosed

---

About This Chapter: Text beginning with the heading "What Is Diabetes?" is excerpted from "Diabetes Overview," National Institute of Diabetes and Digestive and Kidney Diseases (NIDDK), November 2016; Text under the heading "Diabetes And Eating Disorder" is © 2017 Omnigraphics. Reviewed March 2017.

in children and young adults, although it can appear at any age. People with type 1 diabetes need to take insulin every day to stay alive.

Type 2 Diabetes

If you have type 2 diabetes, your body does not make or use insulin well. You can develop type 2 diabetes at any age, even during childhood. However, this type of diabetes occurs most often in middle-aged and older people. Type 2 is the most common type of diabetes.

Gestational Diabetes

Gestational diabetes develops in some women when they are pregnant. Most of the time, this type of diabetes goes away after the baby is born. However, if you've had gestational diabetes, you have a greater chance of developing type 2 diabetes later in life. Sometimes diabetes diagnosed during pregnancy is actually type 2 diabetes.

Other Types Of Diabetes

Less common types include monogenic diabetes, which is an inherited form of diabetes, and cystic fibrosis-related diabetes.

Diabetes Diet And Eating

Nutrition and physical activity are important parts of a healthy lifestyle when you have diabetes. Along with other benefits, following a healthy meal plan and being active can help you keep your blood glucose level, also called blood sugar, in your target range. To manage your blood glucose, you need to balance what you eat and drink with physical activity and diabetes medicine, if you take any. What you choose to eat, how much you eat, and when you eat are all important in keeping your blood glucose level in the range that your healthcare team recommends.

Becoming more active and making changes in what you eat and drink can seem challenging at first. You may find it easier to start with small changes and get help from your family, friends, and healthcare team.

Eating well and being physically active most days of the week can help you:

- keep your blood glucose level, blood pressure, and cholesterol in your target ranges

- lose weight or stay at a healthy weight

- prevent or delay diabetes problems

- feel good and have more energy

What Foods Can I Eat If I Have Diabetes?

You may worry that having diabetes means going without foods you enjoy. The good news is that you can still eat your favorite foods, but you might need to eat smaller portions or enjoy them less often. Your healthcare team will help create a diabetes meal plan for you that meets your needs and likes.

The key to eating with diabetes is to eat a variety of healthy foods from all food groups, in the amounts your meal plan outlines.

The food groups are:

- **vegetables**
  - nonstarchy: includes broccoli, carrots, greens, peppers, and tomatoes
  - starchy: includes potatoes, corn, and green peas
- **fruits**—includes oranges, melon, berries, apples, bananas, and grapes
- **grains**—at least half of your grains for the day should be whole grains
  - includes wheat, rice, oats, cornmeal, barley, and quinoa
  - examples: bread, pasta, cereal, and tortillas
- **protein**
  - lean meat
  - chicken or turkey without the skin
  - fish
  - eggs
  - nuts and peanuts
  - dried beans and certain peas, such as chickpeas and split peas
  - meat substitutes, such as tofu
- **dairy—nonfat or low fat**
  - milk or lactose-free milk if you have lactose intolerance
  - yogurt
  - cheese

Eat foods with heart-healthy fats, which mainly come from these foods:

- oils that are liquid at room temperature, such as canola and olive oil

- nuts and seeds

- heart-healthy fish such as salmon, tuna, and mackerel

- avocado

Use oils when cooking food instead of butter, cream, shortening, lard, or stick margarine.

What Foods And Drinks Should I Limit If I Have Diabetes?

Foods and drinks to limit include:

- fried foods and other foods high in saturated fat and trans fat

- foods high in salt, also called sodium

- sweets, such as baked goods, candy, and ice cream

- beverages with added sugars, such as juice, regular soda, and regular sports or energy drinks

Drink water instead of sweetened beverages. Consider using a sugar substitute in your coffee or tea.

If you drink alcohol, drink moderately—no more than one drink a day if you're a woman or two drinks a day if you're a man. If you use insulin or diabetes medicines that increase the amount of insulin your body makes, alcohol can make your blood glucose level drop too low. This is especially true if you haven't eaten in a while. It's best to eat some food when you drink alcohol.

When Should I Eat If I Have Diabetes?

Some people with diabetes need to eat at about the same time each day. Others can be more flexible with the timing of their meals. Depending on your diabetes medicines or type of insulin, you may need to eat the same amount of carbohydrates at the same time each day. If you take "mealtime" insulin, your eating schedule can be more flexible.

If you use certain diabetes medicines or insulin and you skip or delay a meal, your blood glucose level can drop too low. Ask your healthcare team when you should eat and whether you should eat before and after physical activity.

How Much Can I Eat If I Have Diabetes?

Eating the right amount of food will also help you manage your blood glucose level and your weight. Your healthcare team can help you figure out how much food and how many calories you should eat each day.

Weight-Loss Planning

If you are overweight or obese, work with your healthcare team to create a weight-loss plan.

These tools may help:

- The Body Weight Planner can help you tailor your plans to reach and maintain your goal weight.

- The SuperTracker lets you track your food, physical activity, and weight.

To lose weight, you need to eat fewer calories and replace less healthy foods with foods lower in calories, fat, and sugar.

If you have diabetes, are overweight or obese, and are planning to have a baby, you should try to lose any excess weight before you become pregnant.

Meal Plan Methods

Two common ways to help you plan how much to eat if you have diabetes are the plate method and carbohydrate counting, also called carb counting. Check with your healthcare team about the method that's best for you.

Plate Method

The plate method helps you control your portion sizes. You don't need to count calories. The plate method shows the amount of each food group you should eat. This method works best for lunch and dinner.

Use a 9-inch plate. Put nonstarchy vegetables on half of the plate; a meat or other protein on one-fourth of the plate; and a grain or other starch on the last one-fourth. Starches include starchy vegetables such as corn and peas. You also may eat a small bowl of fruit or a piece of fruit, and drink a small glass of milk as included in your meal plan.

Your daily eating plan also may include small snacks between meals.

Portion Sizes

- You can use everyday objects or your hand to judge the size of a portion.

- 1 serving of meat or poultry is the palm of your hand or a deck of cards

- 1/3-ounce serving of fish is a checkbook

- 1 serving of cheese is six dice

- 1/2 cup of cooked rice or pasta is a rounded handful or a tennis ball

- 1 serving of a pancake or waffle is a DVD

- 2 tablespoons of peanut butter is a ping-pong ball

Carbohydrate Counting

Carbohydrate counting involves keeping track of the amount of carbohydrates you eat and drink each day. Because carbohydrates turn into glucose in your body, they affect your blood glucose level more than other foods do. Carb counting can help you manage your blood glucose level. If you take insulin, counting carbohydrates can help you know how much insulin to take.

The right amount of carbohydrates varies by how you manage your diabetes, including how physically active you are and what medicines you take, if any. Your healthcare team can help you create a personal eating plan based on carbohydrate counting.

The amount of carbohydrates in foods is measured in grams. To count carbohydrate grams in what you eat, you'll need to:

- learn which foods have carbohydrates

- read the Nutrition Facts food label, or learn to estimate the number of grams of carbohydrate in the foods you eat

- add the grams of carbohydrate from each food you eat to get your total for each meal and for the day

Most carbohydrates come from starches, fruits, milk, and sweets. Try to limit carbohydrates with added sugars or those with refined grains, such as white bread and white rice. Instead, eat carbohydrates from fruit, vegetables, whole grains, beans, and low-fat or nonfat milk.

Photo of a bag of groceries containing fruit, vegetables, milk, and bread.

Choose healthy carbohydrates, such as fruit, vegetables, whole grains, beans, and low-fat milk, as part of your diabetes meal plan.

In addition to using the plate method and carb counting, you may want to visit a registered dietitian (RD) for medical nutrition therapy.

What Is Medical Nutrition Therapy?

Medical nutrition therapy is a service provided by an RD to create personal eating plans based on your needs and likes. For people with diabetes, medical nutrition therapy has been shown to improve diabetes management. Medicare pays for medical nutrition therapy for people with diabetes. If you have insurance other than Medicare, ask if it covers medical nutrition therapy for diabetes.

Will Supplements And Vitamins Help My Diabetes?

No clear proof exists that taking dietary supplements such as vitamins, minerals, herbs, or spices can help manage diabetes. You may need supplements if you cannot get enough vitamins and minerals from foods. Talk with your healthcare provider before you take any dietary supplement since some can cause side effects or affect how your medicines work.

Diabetes And Eating Disorders

In individuals suffering from type 1 diabetes, the pancreas is unable to produce insulin, which therefore must be administered daily. A healthy eating plan that balances the periodic insulin injections, physical activity, and food intake is crucial for an individual with this condition. The presence of an eating disorder can cause inadequate glucose control and an increase in the chances of developing secondary complications in the eyes, nerves, and kidneys. In addition to the long-term complications from extreme weight loss, high blood glucose levels induced by omitted or reduced insulin doses can cause diabetic ketoacidosis (DKA), an acidic blood condition that may lead to coma.

Eating disorders that involve episodes of purging or restricting food intake can cause severe low blood sugar (hypoglycemia), which can make it difficult to determine the proper insulin dose for the individual. And those that involve "insulin-purging"—intentionally decreasing insulin dosage as a means of inducing weight loss—may result in a dangerously high blood sugar level (hyperglycemia).

Indications of an eating disorder in a diabetic individual include constant changes in weight, frequent changes in food intake, extreme fear of low blood glucose level (hypoglycemia), anxiety about injecting or injecting in private, and other signs of unusual eating behavior that may not be directly related to diabetes.

Although many diabetic individuals may be prone to developing eating disorders, the risks are higher for adolescents and young women, as the physical and hormonal changes occurring in the body can have an impact on blood sugar levels. It is important for a diabetic individual to seek professional help if even some of these symptoms are present.

Reference

"Eating Disorders and Other Health Problems," Eating Disorders Victoria, June 19, 2015.

Chapter 29

Eating Disorders, Anxiety, And Depression

Psychological conditions like depression and anxiety have been found to co-occur frequently in individuals suffering from eating disorders.

Depression

Depression is a mood disorder that comprises acute feelings of distress, helplessness, anxiety, and/or guilt. It is one of the most common mental-health problems, and it can seriously affect the overall well-being and productivity of the individual.

Symptoms may include:

- Increased frustration

- Insomnia

- Reckless behavior

- Loss of interest in activities that were previously enjoyed

- Irritability

- Feelings of insignificance or self-hatred

- Tendency to abuse alcohol or drugs

- Frequent feelings of fatigue or pain

- Low energy level

"Eating Disorders, Anxiety, And Depression," © 2017 Omnigraphics. Reviewed March 2017.

- Fluctuations in eating habits and body weight
- Social withdrawal
- Poor concentration
- Delusions
- Suicidal thoughts

Depression can be caused by a number of factors, including hormonal imbalance, traumatic experiences, previous history of substance abuse, and side-effects of certain medication. It can either co-occur with, or lead to the development of other mental illnesses, such as anxiety, phobias, panic disorders, and eating disorders.

If You Think You Are Depressed, Ask For Help As Early As You Can

Talk to:

- Your parents or guardian.
- Your teacher or counselor.
- Your doctor.
- A helpline, such as 1-800-273-TALK (8255), free 24-hour help.
- Or call 911 if you are in a crisis or want to hurt yourself.
- Ask your parent or guardian to make an appointment with your doctor for a checkup. Your doctor can make sure that you do not have another health problem that is causing your depression. If your doctor finds that you do not have another health problem, he or she can treat your depression or refer you to a mental health professional. A mental health professional can give you a thorough evaluation and also treat your depression.

(Source: "Teen Depression," National Institute of Mental Health (NIMH).)

It is not clear whether eating disorders take root in an individual due to existing depression, or whether eating disorders cause depression. Since no two eating disorders are the same, and each is a complex condition on its own, both arguments are considered valid in different cases.

For instance, feelings of worthlessness and moodiness are often identified as a sign of an eating disorder, which, on the other hand, may also be symptoms of depression. Likewise, a depressed person can indulge in emotional eating, which can subsequently lead to an eating disorder.

Be Good To Yourself

Besides seeing a doctor and a counselor, you can also help your depression by being patient with yourself and good to yourself. Don't expect to get better immediately, but you will feel yourself improving gradually over time.

- Daily exercise, getting enough sleep, spending time outside in nature and in the sun, or eating healthy foods can also help you feel better.
- Your counselor may teach you how to be aware of your feelings and teach you relaxation techniques. Use these when you start feeling down or upset.
- Try to spend time with supportive family members. Talking with your parents, guardian, or other family members who listen and care about you gives you support and they can make you laugh.
- Try to get out with friends and try fun things that help you express yourself.

(Source: "Teen Depression," National Institute of Mental Health (NIMH).)

Anxiety

It is quite normal for people to feel anxious in stressful situations, but when an individual experiences an extreme and unreasonable level of anxiety, it is characterized as a disorder. Anxiety disorder is generally identified as a combination of psychological states, such as nervousness, fear, worry, and mistrust, that extends over a long period of time and considerably affects daily activities. Anxiety may be caused by a combination of environmental, social, psychological, genetic, and physiological factors.

Some examples include:

- Hormonal imbalance
- Substance abuse, or withdrawal from an illicit drug
- History of mental illness in the family
- Traumatic episodes
- Current physical ailment

Types of anxiety disorders include generalized anxiety disorder (GAD), obsessive-compulsive disorder (OCD), phobias, social anxiety disorder, panic disorder, and posttraumatic stress disorder (PTSD). Each of them has its own unique symptoms, which are further categorized as physical, behavioral, emotional, and cognitive.

Examples Of Different Types Of Anxiety Disorders

- Being very afraid when away from parents (separation anxiety)
- Having extreme fear about a specific thing or situation, such as dogs, insects, or going to the doctor (phobias)
- Being very afraid of school and other places where there are people (social anxiety)
- Being very worried about the future and about bad things happening (general anxiety)
- Having repeated episodes of sudden, unexpected, intense fear that come with symptoms like heart pounding, having trouble breathing, or feeling dizzy, shaky, or sweaty (panic disorder)

(Source: "Anxiety And Depression," Centers for Disease Control and Prevention (CDC).)

Anxiety may present as fear or worry, but can also make children irritable and angry. Anxiety symptoms can also include trouble sleeping, as well as physical symptoms like fatigue, headaches, or stomachaches. Some anxious children keep their worries to themselves and, thus, the symptoms can be missed.

These symptoms include sweating, irregular heartbeat, difficulty in breathing, headache, irregular sleeping patterns, nervous habits, irritability, restlessness, obsessive and unwanted thoughts, and irrational fear.

Like depression, anxiety disorder can co-occur with eating disorders. And similarly, an individual suffering from an anxiety disorder can develop an eating disorder as a means of coping with anxiety. In most cases, anxiety precedes the onset of an eating disorder, such as when an individual briefly soothes symptoms of anxiety by trying to gain a sense of control over other aspects of life, like food, exercise, and weight. This, in the long run, can lead to the development of eating disorders.

Due to the complex nature of eating disorders in conjunction with depression or anxiety, there is the need for an intense treatment plan that analyzes the factors underlying these conditions. Since a number of similar factors can lead to the development of each of these illnesses, successful treatment requires an inclusive strategy that addresses the root cause of all the conditions and helps the individual learn to manage the co-occurring disorder separately and not associate it with food. In addition to medication and nutritional support, the treatment plan may also include various forms of therapy, such as group therapy, cognitive behavioral therapy (CBT), and music and art therapy.

References

1. "Eating Disorders and Other Health Problems," Eating Disorders Victoria, June 19, 2015.

2. Ekern, Jacquelyn. "Dual Diagnosis and Co-Occurring Disorders," Eating Disorder Hope, April 25, 2012

Chapter 30
Eating Disorders And Alcohol And Substance Abuse

The uncontrolled use and abuse of alcohol and drugs can lead to dependence or addiction, which may have severe mental and physical consequences. Alcohol and substance addiction are caused by various biological, social, psychological, environmental, and physiological factors and can co-exist with other medical conditions, as well.

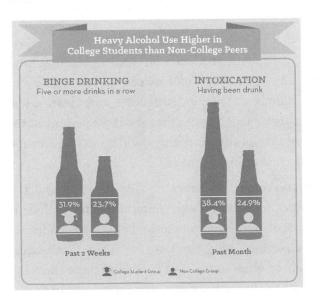

Figure 30.1. Alcohol Usage Among College Students

Source: "Drug and Alcohol Use in College-Age Adults in 2015," National Institute on Drug Abuse.

"Eating Disorders And Alcohol And Substance Abuse," © 2017 Omnigraphics. Reviewed March 2017.

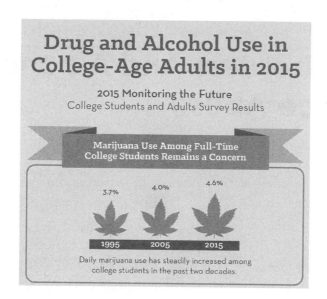

Figure 30.2. Marijuana Usage Among College Students

Source: "Drug and Alcohol Use in College-Age Adults in 2015," National Institute on Drug Abuse.

A three-year study by the National Center on Addiction and Substance Abuse (CASA) at Columbia University showed a strong link between substance abuse and eating disorders—anorexia nervosa and bulimia nervosa, in particular—and identified shared risk factors and characteristics. The exhaustive report states that about 50 percent of those with eating disorders were likely to abuse alcohol and illicit drugs, and up to 35 percent of people with alcohol or drug dependency also had eating disorders.

Other studies have also confirmed that eating disorders and addiction frequently co-occur, noting that characteristics common to both conditions often include intense obsession with the substance (food, alcohol, or drugs), compulsive behavior, a tendency to keep the disorder a secret, social withdrawal, strong cravings, and risk for suicide. Both eating and substance-abuse disorders are more likely to occur in times of stress and depression, low self-esteem, anxiety, when unhealthy dieting behavior or substance abuse is present in the family, and when physical or sexual abuse has occurred in the past.

Both types of disorders are life-threatening, recurrent, and can have the same impact on the functioning of the brain. Some other severe psychiatric conditions associated with eating disorders, as well as substance and alcohol abuse, include obsessive-compulsive disorder and mood disorders.

Eating disorders and alcohol or substance abuse are similar in terms of their addictive nature, and issues related to both conditions tend to coincide. Hence, there is the need for comprehensive treatment that can effectively address the requirements of both disorders simultaneously. Dual-diagnosis treatment and 12-step programs are commonly used in many treatment centers to facilitate eating-disorder and substance-abuse rehabilitation.

Comorbidity

The term "comorbidity" describes two or more disorders or illnesses occurring in the same person. They can occur at the same time or one after the other. Comorbidity also implies interactions between the illnesses that can worsen the course of both.

Many people who are addicted to drugs are also diagnosed with other mental disorders and vice versa. For example, compared with the general population, people addicted to drugs are roughly twice as likely to suffer from mood and anxiety disorders, with the reverse also true.

(Source: Comorbidity: Addiction and Other Mental Disorders. National Institute on Drug Abuse (NIDA))

References

1. "Eating Disorders and Other Health Problems," Eating Disorders Victoria, June 19, 2015.

2. Ekern, Jacquelyn. "Dual Diagnosis and Co-Occurring Disorders," Eating Disorder Hope, April 25, 2012.

Chapter 31

Eating Disorders And Obsessive-Compulsive Disorder

What Is Obsessive-Compulsive Disorder?

Obsessive-compulsive disorder (OCD) is a common, chronic and long-lasting disorder in which a person has uncontrollable, reoccurring thoughts (obsessions) and behaviors (compulsions) that he or she feels the urge to repeat over and over.

Signs And Symptoms

People with OCD may have symptoms of obsessions, compulsions, or both. These symptoms can interfere with all aspects of life, such as work, school, and personal relationships.

Obsessions are repeated thoughts, urges, or mental images that cause anxiety. Common symptoms include:

- Fear of germs or contamination
- Unwanted forbidden or taboo thoughts involving sex, religion, and harm
- Aggressive thoughts towards others or self
- Having things symmetrical or in a perfect order

Compulsions are repetitive behaviors that a person with OCD feels the urge to do in response to an obsessive thought. Common compulsions include:

- Excessive cleaning and/or handwashing

About This Chapter: Text beginning with the heading "What Is Obsessive-Compulsive Disorder?" is excerpted from "Obsessive-Compulsive Disorder," National Institute of Mental Health (NIMH), January 2016; Text under the heading "OCD And Eating Disorders" is © 2017 Omnigraphics. Reviewed March 2017.

- Ordering and arranging things in a particular, precise way

- Repeatedly checking on things, such as repeatedly checking to see if the door is locked or that the oven is off

- Compulsive counting

Not all rituals or habits are compulsions. Everyone double checks things sometimes. But a person with OCD generally:

- Can't control his or her thoughts or behaviors, even when those thoughts or behaviors are recognized as excessive

- Spends at least 1 hour a day on these thoughts or behaviors

- Doesn't get pleasure when performing the behaviors or rituals, but may feel brief relief from the anxiety the thoughts cause

- Experiences significant problems in their daily life due to these thoughts or behaviors

Some individuals with OCD also have a tic disorder. Motor tics are sudden, brief, repetitive movements, such as eye blinking and other eye movements, facial grimacing, shoulder shrugging, and head or shoulder jerking. Common vocal tics include repetitive throat-clearing, sniffing, or grunting sounds.

Symptoms may come and go, ease over time, or worsen. People with OCD may try to help themselves by avoiding situations that trigger their obsessions, or they may use alcohol or drugs to calm themselves. Although most adults with OCD recognize that what they are doing doesn't make sense, some adults and most children may not realize that their behavior is out of the ordinary. Parents or teachers typically recognize OCD symptoms in children.

If you think you have OCD, talk to your doctor about your symptoms. If left untreated, OCD can interfere in all aspects of life.

Risk Factors

OCD is a common disorder that affects adults, adolescents, and children all over the world. Most people are diagnosed by about age 19, typically with an earlier age of onset in boys than in girls, but onset after age 35 does happen. For statistics on OCD in adults, please see the National Institute of Mental Health (NIMH) Obsessive Compulsive Disorder Among Adults webpage.

The causes of OCD are unknown, but risk factors include:

Genetics

Twin and family studies have shown that people with first-degree relatives (such as a parent, sibling, or child) who have OCD are at a higher risk for developing OCD themselves. The risk is higher if the first-degree relative developed OCD as a child or teen. Ongoing research continues to explore the connection between genetics and OCD and may help improve OCD diagnosis and treatment.

Brain Structure And Functioning

Imaging studies have shown differences in the frontal cortex and subcortical structures of the brain in patients with OCD. There appears to be a connection between the OCD symptoms and abnormalities in certain areas of the brain, but that connection is not clear. Research is still underway. Understanding the causes will help determine specific, personalized treatments to treat OCD.

Environment

People who have experienced abuse (physical or sexual) in childhood or other trauma are at an increased risk for developing OCD.

In some cases, children may develop OCD or OCD symptoms following a streptococcal infection—this is called Pediatric Autoimmune Neuropsychiatric Disorders Associated with Streptococcal Infections (PANDAS).

OCD And Eating Disorders

A type of anxiety disorder, obsessive-compulsive disorder (OCD) is characterized by uncontrollable thoughts and repetitive behaviors. The individual often feels anxious and therefore engages in ritualistic or repetitive behaviors to reduce the feeling of uneasiness. OCD often co-occurs with other illnesses, including eating disorders and substance abuse.

Numerous indications of OCD, some more complex than others, may be observed in the behavior of an individual with an eating disorder. Examples include:

- Obsessive thoughts (about food, weight, and body image)

- An obsession with healthy eating and fear of food-borne impurities or diseases (called orthorexia)

- Rituals such as cutting food into tiny pieces or picking food items based on color or shape

- Hoarding large quantities of food

- Spitting out food immediately after chewing

- Excessive or compulsive exercise

These types of abnormal behaviors and thought patterns can take a significant toll on the quality of life, as they can be time-consuming and may create feelings of anxiety and discomfort, especially when in the company of others. Moreover, this situation can lead to a host of other problems, such as depression, irritability, and social isolation.

A strong relationship between eating disorders and OCD has been established, and therefore a comprehensive treatment plan that addresses both forms of illness is crucial. In addition to medication and therapy to treat eating disorders, various forms of psychotherapy may also be employed to bring about a change in the co-occurring unwanted behaviors and thought patterns.

Reference

Ekern, Jacquelyn. "Dual Diagnosis and Co-Occurring Disorders," Eating Disorder Hope, April 25, 2012.

Chapter 32

Eating Disorders And Trichotillomania

Trichotillomania

Trichotillomania is a disorder characterized by an overwhelming urge to repeatedly pull out one's own hair, resulting in hair loss (alopecia). It is classified under the obsessive-compulsive and related disorders category. Trichotillomania results in highly variable patterns of hair loss. The scalp is the most common area of hair pulling, followed by the eyebrows, eyelashes, pubic and perirectal areas, axillae, limbs, torso, and face. The resulting alopecia can range from thin unnoticeable areas of hair loss to total baldness. Some people chew or swallow the hair they pull out (trichophagy), which can result in gastrointestinal problems or develop a trichobezoar (hairball in the intestines or stomach). In many cases, people with this disorder feel extreme tension when they feel an impulse, followed by relief, gratification or pleasure afterwards. The disorder may be mild and manageable, or severe and debilitating. The cause is unknown, though both environmental and genetic causes have been suspected. Treatment may involve cognitive behavior therapy, such as habit reversal training (learning to substitute the hair-pulling behavior) and/or drug therapy, but these are not always effective.

Signs And Symptoms

- Alopecia

- Autosomal dominant inheritance

- Hair-pulling

About This Chapter: Text under the heading "Trichotillomania" is excerpted from "Trichotillomania," Genetic and Rare Diseases Information Center (GARD), March 10, 2017; Text under the heading "Trichotillomania And Eating Disorders," © 2017 Omnigraphics. Reviewed March 2017.

- Multifactorial inheritance

- Obsessive-compulsive behavior

Diagnosis

Making a diagnosis for a genetic or rare disease can often be challenging. Healthcare professionals typically look at a person's medical history, symptoms, physical exam, and laboratory test results in order to make a diagnosis. The following resources provide information relating to diagnosis and testing for this condition. If you have questions about getting a diagnosis, you should contact a healthcare professional.

Testing Resources

- The Genetic Testing Registry (GTR) provides information about the genetic tests for this condition. The intended audience for the GTR is healthcare providers and researchers. Patients and consumers with specific questions about a genetic test should contact a healthcare provider or a genetics professional.

Trichotillomania And Eating Disorders

Current thinking suggests that trichotillomania is most likely caused by multiple factors—genetic, biological, and environmental—and could result in low self-esteem and social withdrawal. Complications include infections, permanent hair loss, and gastrointestinal blockage caused by the ingestion of hair, along with other disorders, such as anxiety, depression, and eating disorders.

Both eating disorders and trichotillomania are often attempts by an individual to cope with negative internal emotions or issues. Obsessive-compulsive behavior is a common trait in both disorders, and the individual suffering from an eating disorder might sense momentary relief when hair is pulled.

Treatment for trichotillomania primarily includes psychotherapy, along with medication and—in some cases—surgery to remove intestinal blockage. A comprehensive treatment method that focuses on resolving underlying issues is usually employed to help the individual heal from both disorders.

Reference

Ekern, Jacquelyn. "Dual Diagnosis and Co-Occurring Disorders," Eating Disorder Hope, April 25, 2012.

Chapter 33

Eating Disorders And Posttraumatic Stress Disorder

Posttraumatic stress disorder (PTSD) develops as a result of exposure to a terrifying or life-threatening event, such as abuse (physical, emotional, or sexual), the sudden death of a loved one, war, major accidents, or natural disasters. The symptoms of PTSD can fall into the following categories:

- **Re-experiencing the traumatic incident.** The individual could have "flashback" episodes, recurring nightmares, and/or reminders or distressing thoughts about the traumatic event, all of which can affect daily life.

- **Avoidance.** The individual may exhibit emotional detachment and avoid people, places, or situations that remind him or her about the event.

- **Stimulation.** These are called arousal symptoms and may include getting alarmed easily, trouble with focusing or sleeping, and sudden emotional outbursts.

- **Negative perceptions and emotions.** These symptoms may include the inability to remember certain parts of the traumatic incident, pessimistic thoughts about people or the world in general, lack of interest in formerly enjoyable activities, and momentary feelings of guilt or blame.

If left untreated, PTSD can have serious adverse effects on the individual. It can take a toll on the person's role in society, interpersonal relationships, the way he or she functions on a daily basis, the ability to learn, and also social and emotional development.

"Eating Disorders And Posttraumatic Stress Disorder," © 2017 Omnigraphics. Reviewed March 2017.

Events Causing PTSD In Children

Any life threatening event or event that threatens physical harm can cause PTSD. These events may include:

- sexual abuse or violence (does not require threat of harm)
- physical abuse
- natural or man made disasters, such as fires, hurricanes, or floods
- violent crimes such as kidnapping or school shootings
- motor vehicle accidents such as automobile and plane crashes

PTSD can also occur after witnessing violence. These events may include exposure to:

- community violence
- domestic violence
- war

Finally, in some cases learning about these events happening to someone close to you can cause PTSD.

(Source: "PTSD In Children And Adolescents," U.S. Department of Veteran Affairs (VA).)

To help cope with the effects of PTSD, individuals frequently develop other disorders, such as drug or alcohol abuse, or an eating disorder. Eating disorders, in particular, have been observed in individuals with a history of trauma, who often perceive this as a way to distract themselves from, or attain a sense of control over, the distressing emotions associated with

What Does PTSD Look Like In Teens?

As in adults, PTSD in children and adolescence requires the presence of re-experiencing, avoidance and numbing, and arousal symptoms. However, researchers and clinicians are beginning to recognize that PTSD may not present itself in children the same way it does in adults. Criteria for PTSD include age-specific features for some symptoms.

PTSD in adolescents may begin to more closely resemble PTSD in adults. However, there are a few features that have been shown to differ. As discussed above, children may engage in traumatic play following a trauma. Adolescents are more likely to engage in traumatic reenactment, in which they incorporate aspects of the trauma into their daily lives. In addition, adolescents are more likely than younger children or adults to exhibit impulsive and aggressive behaviors.

(Source: "PTSD In Children And Adolescents," U.S. Department of Veteran Affairs (VA).)

PTSD. It thus becomes essential to seek help from experienced professionals to treat both conditions simultaneously. A comprehensive treatment strategy may include a combination of medication, nutritional support, and therapy to help resolve the underlying causes of the disorders.

Reference

Ekern, Jacquelyn. "Dual Diagnosis and Co-Occurring Disorders," Eating Disorder Hope, April 25, 2012.

Chapter 34
Could I Have A Mental Health Problem?

Why Do Some People Develop A Mental Health Condition?

Sometimes, people are more at risk because of the genes in their families. Sometimes, people are at risk because of things in their lives, like being abused or using illegal drugs. Sometimes, the cause is something that happened when their moms were pregnant with them, like having a certain virus. For some people, a mix of several things is at work. Whatever the cause, you can get help.

Most of us feel sad, lonely, or anxious at times. That's just human. But sometimes people feel so sad, hopeless, worried, or worthless that they don't want to do things like get out of bed or go to school. These feelings can be signs that you need help for a mental health problem. Depression, anxiety, eating disorders, and other mental health issues can be treated. If you think you have a problem, talk to an adult you trust.

Talk to your parents or a trusted adult if you:

- Can't eat or sleep

- Can't do regular tasks like going to school

- Don't want to do things you used to enjoy

- Don't want to hang out with your friends or family

About This Chapter: This chapter includes text excerpted from "Could I Have A Mental Health Problem?" GirlsHealth.gov, Office on Women's Health (OWH), January 7, 2015.

- Feel like you can't control your feelings and it's hurting your relationships

- Have low energy or no energy

- Feel hopeless

- Feel numb or like nothing matters

- Can't stop thinking about certain things or memories

- Often feel confused or forgetful

- Feel edgy, angry, upset, worried, or scared a lot

- Want to harm yourself or others

- Can't stop yourself from dieting or exercising a lot

- Have aches and pains that don't have a clear cause

- Hear voices

- Feel very sad for months after a loss or death

- Feel like your mind is being controlled or is out of control

Lots of help is available if you are having mental health problems. You can learn about therapy, and you can find a therapist near you. You can text for help with problems and contact a hotline if you're thinking about suicide. Your life can get so much better!

Teens who have faced mental health problems are connecting with each other through photos, videos, and more on OK2TALK.

Online Info

Websites and other online resources sometimes offer great support and tools for mental health. Sometimes, though, they actually promote poor habits. Your best bet is to work with an adult or ask your doctor about any online info.

Chapter 35
Self-Injury And Eating Disorders

Cutting And Self-Harm

Self-harm, sometimes called self-injury, is when a person purposely hurts his or her own body. There are many types of self-injury, and cutting is one type that you may have heard about. If you are hurting yourself, you can learn to stop. Make sure you talk to an adult you trust, and keep reading to learn more.

The Dangers Of Self-Injury

Some teens think self-injury is not a big deal, but it is. Self-injury comes with many risks. For example, cutting can lead to infections, scars, and even death. Sharing tools for cutting puts a person at risk of diseases like human immunodeficiency virus (HIV) and hepatitis. Also, once you start self-injuring, it may be hard to stop. And teens who keep hurting themselves are less likely to learn how to deal with their feelings in healthy ways.

Who Hurts Themselves?

People from all different kinds of backgrounds hurt themselves. Among teens, girls may be more likely to do it than boys.

People of all ages hurt themselves, too, but self-injury most often starts in the teen years.

About This Chapter: Text under the heading "Cutting And Self-Harm" is excerpted from "Cutting And Self-Harm," GirlsHealth.gov, Office on Women's Health (OWH), January 7, 2015; Text under the heading "Self-Injury And Eating Disorders," is © 2017 Omnigraphics. Reviewed March 2017.

People who hurt themselves sometimes have other problems like depression, eating disorders, or drug or alcohol abuse.

Why Do Some Teens Hurt Themselves?

Some teens who hurt themselves keep their feelings bottled up inside. The physical pain then offers a sense of relief, like the feelings are getting out. Some people who hold back strong emotions begin to feel like they have no emotions, and the injury helps them at least feel something.

Some teens say that when they hurt themselves, they are trying to stop feeling painful emotions, like rage, loneliness, or hopelessness. They may injure to distract themselves from the emotional pain. Or they may be trying to feel some sense of control over what they feel.

If you are depressed, angry, or having a hard time coping, talk with an adult you trust. You also can contact a helpline. Remember, you have a right to be safe and happy!

If you are hurting yourself, please get help. It is possible to get past the urge to hurt yourself. There are other ways to deal with your feelings. You can talk to your parents, your doctor, or another trusted adult, like a teacher or religious leader. Therapy can help you find healthy ways to handle problems.

What Are Signs Of Self-Injury In Others?

- Having cuts, bruises, or scars
- Wearing long sleeves or pants even in hot weather
- Making excuses about injuries
- Having sharp objects around for no clear reason

How Can I Help A Friend Who Is Self-Injuring?

If you think a friend may be hurting herself, try to get your friend to talk to a trusted adult. Your friend may need professional help. A therapist can suggest ways to cope with problems without turning to self-injury. If your friend won't get help, you should talk to an adult. This is too much for you to handle alone.

What If Someone Pressures Me To Hurt Myself?

If someone pressures you to hurt yourself, think about whether you really want a friend who tries to cause you pain. Try to hang out with other people who don't treat you this way. Try to hang out with people who make you feel good about yourself.

Eating Disorders And Self-Injury

The likelihood of engaging in self-injury is high for individuals with eating disorders. Similarly, certain behaviors associated with eating disorders—such as induced vomiting, excessive or compulsive exercise, and excessive consumption of laxatives—can be the cause self-harm.

And self-injury could, alternatively, act as a means of expressing dissatisfaction with one's body, punishing oneself for not sticking to a routine, or even finding solace from a strict nutritional regimen. During the diagnosis and treatment of eating disorders, identifying the signs of self-harm, as well as analyzing its causes, are essential for a successful outcome. Medication, along with various forms of psychotherapy, such as family intervention, group therapy, and cognitive-behavioral therapy (CBT), will aid in faster recovery from both eating disorders and self-injurious behavior.

Common forms of self-injury include cutting skin, scratching, beating or burning body parts, interfering with the healing of wounds, and the intake of poisonous substances. Self-injury can be caused by a combination of psychological, genetic, and social factors, along with a possible history of substance abuse and other destructive behavior. Rarely does an individual engage in self-harm with the intention of committing suicide, but these habits, if left unchecked, can increase the risk of death.

The reasons for self-injury can include establishing a sense of control, relieving negative emotions (such as anger, shame, distress, guilt, or loneliness), and attempting to escape traumatic memories. The consequences and complications of such behaviors may include depression, poor self-esteem, relationship difficulties, infections, hospitalization, or even death.

Self-injury and suicidal thoughts are compulsive behaviors that can also manifest as a co-occurring disorder. Signs of self-injury, such as fresh wounds, multiple scars, frequent withdrawal from friends and family, and covering wounds with long sleeves or pants, could be an indication of the presence of another illness.

Reference

Ekern, Jacquelyn. "Dual Diagnosis and Co-Occurring Disorders," Eating Disorder Hope, April 25, 2012.

Part Four
Diagnosing And Treating Eating Disorders

Chapter 36

Common Symptoms Of Eating Disorders

There is a commonly held view that eating disorders are a lifestyle choice. Eating disorders are actually serious and often fatal illnesses that cause severe disturbances to a person's eating behaviors. Obsessions with food, body weight, and shape may also signal an eating disorder. Common eating disorders include anorexia nervosa, bulimia nervosa, and binge eating disorder.

Fast Fact

Eating disorders can start at any age, but they usually start during the teen years. Females are more likely to get eating disorders than males.

(Source: "Having Eating Disorders," Office on Women's Health (OWH), U.S. Department of Health and Human Services (HHS).)

Anorexia Nervosa

People with anorexia nervosa may see themselves as overweight, even when they are dangerously underweight. People with anorexia nervosa typically weigh themselves repeatedly, severely restrict the amount of food they eat, and eat very small quantities of only certain foods. Anorexia nervosa has the highest mortality rate of any mental disorder. While many young women and men with this disorder die from complications associated with starvation, others

---

About This Chapter: This chapter includes text excerpted from "Eating Disorders," National Institute of Mental Health (NIMH), February 2016.

die of suicide. In women, suicide is much more common in those with anorexia than with most other mental disorders.

Symptoms include:

- Extremely restricted eating

- Extreme thinness (emaciation)

- A relentless pursuit of thinness and unwillingness to maintain a normal or healthy weight

- Intense fear of gaining weight

- Distorted body image, a self-esteem that is heavily influenced by perceptions of body weight and shape, or a denial of the seriousness of low body weight

Other symptoms may develop over time, including:

- Thinning of the bones (osteopenia or osteoporosis)

- Mild anemia and muscle wasting and weakness

- Brittle hair and nails

- Dry and yellowish skin

- Growth of fine hair all over the body (lanugo)

- Severe constipation

- Low blood pressure, slowed breathing and pulse

- Damage to the structure and function of the heart

- Brain damage

- Multiorgan failure

- Drop in internal body temperature, causing a person to feel cold all the time

- Lethargy, sluggishness, or feeling tired all the time

- Infertility

Bulimia Nervosa

People with bulimia nervosa have recurrent and frequent episodes of eating unusually large amounts of food and feeling a lack of control over these episodes. This binge-eating is followed by behavior that compensates for the overeating such as forced vomiting, excessive use of laxatives or diuretics, fasting, excessive exercise, or a combination of these behaviors. Unlike anorexia nervosa, people with bulimia nervosa usually maintain what is considered a healthy or relatively normal weight.

Symptoms include:

- Chronically inflamed and sore throat

- Swollen salivary glands in the neck and jaw area

- Worn tooth enamel and increasingly sensitive and decaying teeth as a result of exposure to stomach acid

- Acid reflux disorder and other gastrointestinal problems

- Intestinal distress and irritation from laxative abuse

- Severe dehydration from purging of fluids

- Electrolyte imbalance (too low or too high levels of sodium, calcium, potassium and other minerals) which can lead to stroke or heart attack

---

Trying to make up for the binging can take different forms. Some examples include the following:

- Purging, which means trying to get rid of the food. This could include:
- Making yourself throw up
- Taking laxatives (pills or liquids that cause a bowel movement)
- Exercising a lot
- Eating very little or not at all
- Taking pills to urinate (pee) often to lose weight

(Source: "Having Eating Disorders," Office on Women's Health (OWH), U.S. Department of Health and Human Services (HHS).)

Chapter 37

When You Suspect Someone You Know Has An Eating Disorder

How To Help A Friend With Eating And Body Image Issues

If you are reading this, chances are you are concerned about the eating habits, weight, or body image of someone you care about. We understand that this can be a very difficult and scary time for you. Let us assure you that you are doing a great thing by looking for more information! This list may not tell you everything you need to know about what to do in your specific situation, but it will give you some helpful ideas on what to do to help your friend.

Learn as much as you can about eating disorders. Read books, articles, and brochures.

Know the difference between facts and myths about weight, nutrition, and exercise. Knowing the facts will help you reason with your friend about any inaccurate ideas that may be fueling their disordered eating patterns.

Be honest. Talk openly and honestly about your concerns with the person who is struggling with eating or body image problems. Avoiding it or ignoring it won't help!

Be caring, but be firm. Caring about your friend does not mean being manipulated by them. Your friend must be responsible for their actions and the consequences of those actions. Avoid making rules, promises, or expectations that you cannot or will not uphold. For example, "I promise not to tell anyone." Or, "If you do this one more time, I'll never talk to you again."

Compliment your friend's wonderful personality, successes, or accomplishments. Remind your friend that "true beauty" is not skin deep.

About This Chapter: Text in this chapter is excerpted from "For Family And Friends," © 2016 National Eating Disorders Association. For more information, visit www.nationaleatingdisorders.org. Reprinted with permission.

Be a good role model in regard to sensible eating, exercise, and self-acceptance.

Tell someone. It may seem difficult to know when, if at all, to tell someone else about your concerns. Addressing body image or eating problems in their beginning stages offers your friend the best chance for working through these issues and becoming healthy again. Don't wait until the situation is so severe that your friend's life is in danger. Your friend needs a great deal of support and understanding.

Remember that you cannot force someone to seek help, change their habits, or adjust their attitudes. You can make important progress in honestly sharing your concerns, providing support, and knowing where to go for more information! **People struggling with anorexia, bulimia, or binge eating disorder do need professional help.**

What Should I Say?

Tips For Talking To A Friend Who May Be Struggling With An Eating Disorder

If you are worried about your friend's eating behaviors or attitudes, it is important to express your concerns in a loving and supportive way. It is also necessary to discuss your worries early on, rather than waiting until your friend has endured many of the damaging physical and emotional effects of eating disorders. In a private and relaxed setting, talk to your friend in a calm and caring way about the specific things you have seen or felt that have caused you to worry.

What To Say—Step By Step

Set a time to talk. Set aside a time for a private, respectful meeting with your friend to discuss your concerns openly and honestly in a caring, supportive way. Make sure you will be some place away from distractions.

Communicate your concerns. Share your memories of specific times when you felt concerned about your friend's eating or exercise behaviors. Explain that you think these things may indicate that there could be a problem that needs professional attention.

Ask your friend to explore these concerns with a counselor, doctor, nutritionist, or other health professional who is knowledgeable about eating disorders. If you feel comfortable doing so, offer to help your friend make an appointment or accompany your friend on their first visit.

Avoid conflicts or a battle of wills with your friend. If your friend refuses to acknowledge that there is a problem, or any reason for you to be concerned, restate your feelings and the reasons for them and leave yourself open and available as a supportive listener.

Avoid placing shame, blame, or guilt on your friend regarding their actions or attitudes. Do not use accusatory "you" statements such as, "You just need to eat." Or, "You are acting irresponsibly." Instead, use "I" statements. For example: "I'm concerned about you because you refuse to eat breakfast or lunch." Or, "It makes me afraid to hear you vomiting."

Avoid giving simple solutions. For example, "If you'd just stop, then everything would be fine!"

Express your continued support. Remind your friend that you care and want your friend to be healthy and happy.

After talking with your friend, if you are still concerned with their health and safety, **find a trusted adult or medical professional to talk to.** This is probably a challenging time for both of you. It could be helpful for you, as well as your friend, to discuss your concerns and seek assistance and support from a professional.

Chapter 38
Diagnosing Eating Disorders

Little is known about ideal screening for eating disorders (EDs) in substance use disorder (SUD) treatment programs. Researchers recommend that SUD treatment programs screen for EDs, along with other behavioral health disorders, at intake and intermittently during treatment of all patients in SUD treatment. An analysis of National Treatment Center Study data notes that programs that screen for EDs do so during intake and assessment.

About half these programs screen all admissions for EDs, and half screen only when an ED is suspected. Screening for EDs only when one is suspected can be complex, because signs and symptoms of EDs can overlap with those of SUDs or with those of other behavioral health problems. For example, weight loss, lethargy, changes in eating habits, and depressed mood can indicate an SUD or an affective disorder. In addition, signs may not be readily observable to counselors, because people with EDs often go to great lengths to disguise and hide their disorder. However, counselors should be aware of common red flags for EDs that tend not to overlap with those of other behavioral health disorders. Given below are some indications (in addition to Diagnostic and Statistical Manual of Mental Disorders (DSM) criteria) that an ED may be present.

Screening for EDs will likely result in identification for the need of further assessment and treatment. SUD treatment counselors can easily (and unobtrusively) incorporate some ED screening into the SUD assessment in a number of ways:

- As part of the drug use assessment patients should provide information about their use of over-the-counter and prescription laxatives, diuretics, and diet pills.

About This Chapter: This chapter includes text excerpted from "Clients With Substance Use And Eating Disorders," Substance Abuse and Mental Health Services Administration (SAMHSA), February 2011. Reviewed March 2017.

- As part of taking a medical history, patients are asked about past hospitalizations and behavioral health treatment history, including for EDs.

- As part of assessing daily activities, patients are asked how often and for how long they exercise.

- Patients are asked, "Other than those we've discussed so far, are there any health issues that concern you?"

Body Mass Index (BMI)

BMI is a number derived from a calculation based on a person's weight and height. For most people, BMI correlates with their amount of body fat. Measuring BMI is an inexpensive and easy alternative to a direct measurement of body fat percentage and is a useful method of screening for weight categories that may lead to health problems. BMI categories are:

- Underweight: BMI score of less than 18.5

Table 38.1. BMI Score For Underweight

Severe thinness	BMI score of less than 16
Moderate thinness	BMI score between 16.00 and 16.99
Mild thinness	BMI score between 17.00 and 18.49

- Normal range: BMI score between 18.5 and 24.9

- Overweight: BMI score between 25.0 and 29.9

- Obese: BMI score of 30.0 or more

BMI in children and adolescents is calculated somewhat differently from BMI in adults.

Severe thinness	BMI score of less than 16
Moderate thinness	BMI score between 16.00 and 16.99
Mild thinness	BMI score between 17.00 and 18.49

DSM-IV-TR Diagnostic Criteria For Anorexia Nervosa

- Refusal to maintain body weight at or above a minimally normal weight for age and height (e.g., weight loss leading to maintenance of body weight less than 85 percent of that expected; or failure to make expected weight gain during period of growth, leading to body weight less than 85 percent of that expected).

- Intense fear of gaining weight or becoming fat, even though underweight.

- Disturbance in the way in which one's body weight or shape is experienced, undue influence of body weight or shape on self-evaluation, or denial of the seriousness of the current low body weight.

- In postmenarcheal females, amenorrhea, i.e., the absence of at least three consecutive menstrual cycles. (A woman is considered to have amenorrhea if her periods only occur following hormone therapies, e.g., estrogen administration.)

DSM-IV-TR Diagnostic Criteria For Bulimia Nervosa

- Recurrent episodes of binge eating. An episode of binge eating is characterized by both of the following:

  - Eating, in a discrete period of time (e.g., within any 2-hour period), an amount of food that is definitely larger than most people would eat during a similar period of time and under similar circumstances

  - A sense of lack of control overeating during the episode (e.g., a feeling that one cannot stop eating or control what or how much one is eating)

- Recurrent inappropriate compensatory behavior in order to prevent weight gain, such as self-induced vomiting; misuse of laxatives, diuretics, enemas, or other medications; fasting; or excessive exercise.

- The binge eating and inappropriate compensatory behaviors both occur, on average, at least twice a week for 3 months.

- Self-evaluation is unduly influenced by body shape and weight.

- The disturbance does not occur exclusively during episodes of anorexia nervosa.

Proposed DSM-5 Diagnostic Criteria For Binge Eating Disorder

- Recurrent episodes of binge eating. An episode of binge eating is characterized by both of the following:

  - Eating, in a discrete period of time (for example, within any 2-hour period), an amount of food that is definitely larger than most people would eat in a similar period of time under similar circumstances

  - A sense of lack of control overeating during the episode (for example, a feeling that one cannot stop eating or control what or how much one is eating)

- The binge eating episodes are associated with three (or more) of the following:
  - Eating much more rapidly than normal
  - Eating until feeling uncomfortably full
  - Eating large amounts of food when not feeling physically hungry
  - Eating alone because of being embarrassed by how much one is eating
  - Feeling disgusted with oneself, depressed, or very guilty afterwards
- Marked distress regarding binge eating is present.
- The binge eating occurs, on average, at least once a week for three months.
- The binge eating is not associated with the recurrent use of inappropriate compensatory behavior (for example, purging) and does not occur exclusively during the course of anorexia nervosa, bulimia nervosa, or avoidant/restrictive food intake disorder.

Chapter 39
Going To Therapy

Lots of teens have some kind of emotional problem. In fact, almost half of U.S. teens will have a mental health problem before they turn 18. The good news is that therapy can really help.

Sometimes, people are embarrassed or afraid to see a therapist. But getting help from a therapist because you're feeling sad or anxious is really not different from seeing a doctor because you broke a bone. In fact, you can feel proud for being brave enough to do what you need to do to get your life back on track.

What Is Therapy?

Therapy is when you talk about your problems with someone who is a professional counselor, such as a psychiatrist, psychologist, or social worker. Therapy sometimes is called psychotherapy. That is because it helps with your psychology—the mental and emotional parts of your life.

If you are going through a rough time, talking to a caring therapist can be a great relief. A therapist can help you cope with sadness, worry, and other strong or scary feelings. Here are some other ways therapy can help:

- It can teach you specific skills for handling difficult situations, such as problems with your family or school.

- It can help you find healthy ways to deal with stress or anger.

- It can teach you how to build healthy relationships.

About This Chapter: This chapter includes text excerpted from "Going To Therapy," GirlsHealth.gov, Office on Women's Health (OWH), January 7, 2015.

- It can help you figure out how to think about things in more positive ways.

- It can help you figure out how to boost your self-confidence.

- It can help you decide where you want to go in life and how to deal with any obstacles that may come up along the way.

Therapy may feel great right away, or it might feel strange at first. It can take a little time getting used to talking with someone new about your problems. But therapists are trained to listen well, and they want to help.

As time goes on, you should feel comfortable with your therapist. If you don't feel comfortable, or if you think you're not getting better, tell your parent or guardian. Another therapist or type of therapy might work better.

Therapists protect people's privacy. They can share what you say only in very special cases, such as if they think you are in danger. If you're concerned, though, ask about the privacy policy. It's important to feel like you can tell the truth in therapy. It works best if you are honest about any problems you're facing, including problems with drugs or alcohol or any behaviors that can hurt your body or mind.

Just because you start to see a therapist doesn't mean that you will see one forever. You should be able to learn skills that let you handle your problems on your own. Sometimes, a few sessions are all you need to learn skills and feel better.

Want to know more about therapy? You can get more info on seeing a therapist, including whether or not to tell your friends.

Why Do Teens Go For Therapy?

Many young people develop mental health conditions, like depression, eating disorders, or anxiety disorders. If you have a mental health problem, remember there are treatments that work, and you can feel better. Also, some teens go to therapy to get help through a tough time, like their parents' getting divorced or having too much stress at school.

If you feel out of control, or you feel like a mental health problem keeps you from enjoying life, get help. Reach out to a parent or guardian or another trusted adult.

What Should I Do To Get Started With Therapy?

If you need help finding a therapist, you can start by talking to your doctor, school nurse, or school counselor. If your family has insurance, the insurance company can tell you which therapists are covered under your plan. You and your parent or guardian also can look online for mental health treatment.

If you need help paying for therapy, you can ask a parent or guardian if they have health insurance that might help pay for therapy. If your family doesn't have insurance, they can find out about getting it through healthcare.gov. You also may be able to get free or low-cost therapy at a mental health clinic, hospital, university, or other places.

What Are Some Kinds Of Therapy?

There are different kinds of therapy to help you feel better. The best treatment depends on the type of problem that you are facing.

You may have one-on-one talk therapy. This is when you talk to a therapist alone. Or you may join group therapy, where you work with a therapist and other people who are having similar issues. You may also do art therapy, where you paint or draw.

One kind of talk therapy that tends to work well for depression, anxiety, and several other problems is cognitive behavioral therapy. This type of therapy teaches you how to think and act in healthier ways.

Sometimes, your therapist will suggest that you take medicine in addition to therapy, which often can be a helpful combination.

What About Online Support Groups?

There are lots of support groups available on the Internet, including ones to help you handle your feelings. Chat rooms and other online options may help you feel less alone. But if you are having trouble coping, it's important to work with a therapist or other mental health professional.

Remember to be careful about getting info online. Some people use the Internet to promote unhealthy behaviors, like cutting and dangerous eating habits.

Chapter 40
Treating Eating Disorders

How Do I Get Help For Eating Disorders?

Eating disorders are real medical illnesses. They can lead to serious problems with your heart and other parts of your body. They even can lead to death.

Eating disorders are treatable. Girls with eating disorders can go on to lead full, happy lives.

Treatment for an eating disorder may include talk therapy, medicine, and nutrition counseling. Treatment depends on the type of disorder and the needs of the person who has it.

If you think you have an eating disorder, talk to your doctor or another trusted adult. You also can call or chat with a special eating disorders helpline. Sometimes, a person doesn't have an eating disorder, but has unhealthy dieting behaviors that can turn into an eating disorder. If that's you, get help before any problems get worse. You deserve to feel great!

If you have an eating disorder, you may feel really bad. Don't give up! You can feel better.

> ### Eating Disorder Recovery
> Confronting the eating disorder is the first step of eating disorder recovery. If you are suffering with an eating disorder, it is important to admit that you need help.

About This Chapter: Text under the heading "How Do I Get Help For Eating Disorders?" is excerpted from "Having Eating Disorders," GirlsHealth.gov, Office on Women's Health (OWH), January 7, 2015; Text under the heading "Treatments And Therapies" is excerpted from "Eating Disorders," National Institute of Mental Health (NIMH), February 2016.

Treatments And Therapies

Adequate nutrition, reducing excessive exercise, and stopping purging behaviors are the foundations of treatment. Treatment plans are tailored to individual needs and may include one or more of the following:

- Individual, group, and/or family psychotherapy
- Medications

Psychotherapies

Psychotherapies such as a family-based therapy called the Maudsley approach, where parents of adolescents with anorexia nervosa assume responsibility for feeding their child, appear to be very effective in helping people gain weight and improve eating habits and moods.

To reduce or eliminate binge-eating and purging behaviors, people may undergo cognitive behavioral therapy (CBT), which is another type of psychotherapy that helps a person learn how to identify distorted or unhelpful thinking patterns and recognize and change inaccurate beliefs.

Medical Nutrition Therapy (MNT)

Medical Nutrition Therapy (MNT) is a holistic and therapeutic method for treating medical conditions and correlating symptoms. It is used to treat an illness or condition, or as a means to prevent or delay disease or complications from diseases such as diabetes. Medical Nutrition Therapy is established on the idea that several medical conditions progress or are made worse by an inadequate diet or insufficient nutrient intake.

Medications

Evidence also suggests that medications such as antidepressants, antipsychotics, or mood stabilizers approved by the U.S. Food and Drug Administration (FDA) may also be helpful for treating eating disorders and other co-occurring illnesses such as anxiety or depression.

What Is Being Done To Better Understand And Treat Eating Disorders?

Researchers are finding that eating disorders are caused by a complex interaction of genetic, biological, psychological, and social factors. But many questions still need answers. Researchers are studying questions about behavior, genetics, and brain function to better understand risk factors, identify biological markers, and develop specific psychotherapies and medications that can target areas in the brain that control eating behavior. Brain imaging and genetic studies may provide clues for how each person may respond to specific treatments for these medical illnesses. Ongoing efforts also are aimed at developing and refining strategies for preventing and treating eating disorders among adolescents and adults.

(Source: "Eating Disorders: About More Than Food," National Institute of Mental Health (NIMH).)

Chapter 41

Types Of Therapy For Eating Disorder

Eating disorders are health conditions with serious physical, psychological, and social consequences. What starts out as an urge to eat less or more in response to a distorted perception of body image, may spiral out of control and become a debilitating or chronic medical illness. Early intervention is key to successful treatment outcomes and may avoid the fatal or life-threatening conditions often associated with eating disorders, such as anorexia nervosa. Studies have shown that multiple factors—genetic, biological, psychological, and social—determine the cause of eating disorders, and efforts are underway to develop specific psychotherapies and medications that can control eating behavior by targeting specific centers in the brain.

Treating Eating Disorders

Treatment may include therapy to help you change your eating habits, as well as thoughts and feelings that may lead to binge eating and other psychological symptoms. Types of therapy that have been shown to help people with binge eating disorder are called psychotherapies and include cognitive behavioral therapy, interpersonal psychotherapy, and dialectical behavior therapy. Your psychiatrist or other healthcare provider may also prescribe medication to help you with your binge eating, or to treat other medical or mental health problems.

(Source: "Diagnosis And Treatment Of Binge Eating Disorder," National Institute of Diabetes and Digestive and Kidney Diseases (NIDDK).)

Typically, treatment goals involve formulating a healthy nutrition plan, restoring body weight to a prescribed level, and stopping such behaviors as binge eating and purging.

"Types Of Therapy," © 2017 Omnigraphics. Reviewed March 2017.

Treatment plans are tailored to meet individual requirements and also treat co-existing conditions, such as depression, substance abuse, or personality disorders. While some types of psychotherapy can be provided on an outpatient basis, others may require hospitalization to treat the more severe effects of malnutrition.

The treatment protocol for eating disorders is highly dependent on the type and severity of the disorder and any associated conditions. It may include one or a combination of the following:

- Individual, family, or group psychotherapy

- Medical care and monitoring

- Nutritional counseling

- Medications (for example, antidepressants)

Some Common Types Of Therapy Available For Eating Disorders

Cognitive Behavioral Therapy (CBT)

CBT is one of the most widely practiced forms of psychological intervention for treating eating disorders. Developed by psychotherapist Aaron Beck, M.D., in the 1960s, CBT combines two therapies, cognitive therapy (CT) and behavioral therapy, and is based on the theory that negative thoughts and negative behavior are interlinked. This kind of therapy focuses on helping individuals recognize the irrational thinking patterns associated with food and body image, then develop positive and healthy behavior patterns.

The treatment plan usually includes three phases and requires the active participation of both patient and therapist. The first phase is called the behavioral phase, in which the therapist and the patient devise a plan to stabilize eating behavior, treat symptoms, and learn coping mechanisms with the help of in-session activities. The second phase, the cognitive phase, involves restructuring techniques intended to change harmful and problematic thinking patterns and replace them with new perspectives and ideas. This phase also assesses other psychological and social factors, such as relationship problems or low self-esteem, that may underlie the eating problem. The final phase of CBT is the relapse prevention phase. Here the focus is on eliminating triggers and maintaining the progress made thus far. CBT is almost always incorporated into the treatment plan for eating disorders because of its adaptability in creating individualized therapy to achieve personal goals and promote holistic healing.

Medical Nutrition Therapy (MNT)

This type of treatment, an essential part of the treatment plan for eating disorders, focuses on helping patients normalize their eating patterns. Creating a healthy eating regimen includes maintaining a nutritious and balanced diet, promoting a harmonious and sustainable relationship with food devoid of negative or harmful rationale, and learning to trust the body's natural response to feelings of hunger or fullness.

MNT can be implemented in all kinds of treatment settings, including inpatient, outpatient, and residential care facilities. In all cases, a registered dietician formulates a structured meal plan on the basis of the patient's medical history, as well as his or her dietary and laboratory evaluations, and supervises the implementation of the dietary plan. The dietitian also educates the patient on the importance of following the prescribed diet plan and avoiding dysfunctional eating behavior and may also modify the plan to address specific deficiencies or medical conditions.

Dialectical Behavioral Therapy (DBT)

Dialectical behavior therapy is a form of CBT originally developed to treat people with borderline personality disorder. The term "dialectical" refers to a discussion that takes place between two people holding opposing views until they find common ground or achieve a balance between the two extreme views. In a treatment setting, the therapist engages in a philosophical exercise with the patient and tries to make him or her responsible for disruptive behavior, while at the same time assuring the patient that illogical thoughts and actions are understandable and not necessarily destructive.

In recent years, DBT has often been incorporated into treatment plans for eating disorders—in both individual and group therapy sessions—and is known to have better outcomes than CBT, which is based more on the premise that the patient's thoughts have to be controlled or changed. In contrast, DBT is based more on acceptance of the patient's extreme behavior and gradual progress toward recognizing triggers, learning to perceive when boundaries are overstepped, and acquiring skills to deal with conflict and stress.

This form of psychotherapy accepts the fact that the patient has spent months—even years—developing eating-disorder patterns and would find it difficult to switch them off in a day. For instance, an anorexic's "I am fat" mindset is not something he or she can unlearn quickly, but developing a heightened awareness of thought processes can help control negative emotions and shift focus to healthy and positive emotions. DBT relies greatly on a close relationship between patient and therapist, and while patients learn new skills during individual sessions, they get an opportunity to practice their newly acquired skills at group sessions.

Expressive Or Creative Arts Therapy

Expressive or creative arts therapy uses the creative process to help people treat depression and eating disorders. Used in conjunction with other traditional therapies, this approach has been particularly beneficial in people with a history of trauma.

Art therapy is based on developing self-awareness and centers on the experiences and perceptions of the individual. The process of creating an image of one's thoughts, emotions, and conflicts through the medium of art—say sculpting or painting—is often called "concretization.," which can help the patient accept and recognize his or her inner self-through the use of symbols. These symbols of self-expression may also help the therapist in diagnosis, in addition to providing research material for this relatively new field.

Art provides a creative outlet for self-expression and offers a coping mechanism for self-destructive behavior, such as bingeing or purging. A licensed creative-arts therapist can assess, evaluate, and provide therapeutic intervention for the treatment of eating disorders through the use of such activities as drawing, painting, sculpting, photography, music, dance, and drama.

Animal-Assisted Therapy

Although early studies have shown that companion animals contribute significantly to mental and emotional well-being, it is only recently that animal-assisted therapy has begun to be used in conjunction with established therapies to treat many types of mental disorders. Working or playing with animals, such as cats, dogs, or horses, is increasingly being incorporated into the treatment of behavioral problems, particularly in pediatric settings.

For example, equine-assisted psychotherapy is being used as an effective treatment for such disorders as anxiety, attention deficit hyperactivity disorder (ADHD), depression, eating disorders, and posttraumatic stress disorder (PTSD). Caring for animals has been shown to improve self-image in people with eating disorders, and patients also forge an emotional bond with animals, which provides them with a means of self-expression while also teaching them coping mechanisms to deal with self-injurious thoughts and emotions.

Play Therapy

Play therapy is commonly used as a therapeutic intervention, particularly in children and adolescents, as it provides them with an opportunity to express and communicate at their own pace. Toys and games help children make developmentally appropriate responses and also allows the therapist to gain insight into the child's inner world.

Studies have shown that each child's personal experience plays a role in determining the child's self-image as well as the behavioral tendencies that he or she develops to function in the world. Play therapy helps focus on the child's effort to develop coping mechanisms to resolve social or emotional conflict, both in the present and the future. More recently, play therapy has gained momentum as an effective treatment tool for behavioral disorders, including binge-eating and anorexia nervosa, as it offers a safe environment in which children can work toward finding their sense of emotional stability without having to relive past traumas.

Family-Based Therapy

Family-based therapy was developed from the premise that involving family and improving relationships between family members increases the likelihood of a positive treatment outcome. Therapists work at resolving conflicts within the family, educating relatives about the patient's condition and early signs of problems, and charting out an action plan to manage the condition effectively.

Studies have shown favorable outcomes with family-focused therapy in terms of both stabilizing treatment and preventing relapse. Moreover, this kind of therapy builds better understanding and communication and has been effective in preventing "burn out" in family caregivers, which could in turn result in apathy to the patient's condition.

The Maudsley Approach

One type of family-based therapy, called the Maudsley approach for its development at Maudsley Hospital in London, has proven to be effective in the long-term improvement of anorexia nervosa and bulimia nervosa, particularly in adolescents. This approach is characterized by three distinct procedural stages:

- Weight restoration
- Returning control overeating to the teen
- Establishing healthy adolescent identity

In the first phase, the parents are made responsible for helping the teen adopt a healthy eating plan. They are also counseled on the child's condition and how to refrain from criticism. The second phase involves getting the patient to assume responsibility for his or her eating habits. Here, there is a gradual shift away from parental control, and the patient is encouraged to develop the cognitive processes required to take responsibility for healthy nutrition. The third stage begins after the patient reaches and maintains a healthy body weight. During this stage, the therapist helps the patient develop a healthy identity and resolve adolescent and family issues that may underlie the eating disorder. The therapist also helps the patient develop autonomy while helping caregivers cope with high anxiety and stress, which may be counter-productive to the success of family-based therapies.

Despite this method gaining popularity as a treatment regime for binge eating and anorexia, Maudsley studies have shown that the model has had mixed outcomes with older adolescents, adults, and the chronically ill. Moreover, the high degree of parental involvement in the treatment and recovery process may sometimes further exacerbate dysfunctional patterns in adolescents and make it difficult for the patient to gain autonomy, something crucial to the recovery phase. And yet, notwithstanding these issues, the Maudsley approach continues to be a popular therapeutic modality studied by researchers across the United States and Europe.

Phototherapy

Bright light therapy has traditionally been used in the treatment of seasonal affective disorder (SAD), a form of depression associated with imbalances of melatonin, a hormone that regulates the sleep and wake cycles, often referred to as the circadian rhythm. SAD may also be attributed to a fall in the levels of serotonin, a neurotransmitter responsible for maintaining mood, sleep and appetite.

Melatonin is produced nocturnally by the **pineal gland,** and its production stops with exposure to sunlight. It has been proven that exposure to bright light or natural sunlight during the day triggers early nocturnal production of melatonin, thereby enhancing sleep cycle, appetite, and mood. Serotonin is a precursor of melatonin and is also influenced by sunlight. Although it is produced during the day, the conversion of serotonin to melatonin occurs at night. Short days and long nights in winter not only lower serotonin production during the day, but also causes delayed nighttime melatonin production, both of which negatively impact energy levels, sleep, and sense of well-being.

Light therapy is administered by exposing the patient to bright light for prescribed periods of time. In recent years, light therapy has been used to treat eating disorders, in conjunction with other established therapies. Disorders such as bulimia nervosa or binge eating share certain features with SAD, in that symptoms are seasonal and depression is a coexisting condition. Although more studies are needed before drawing definitive conclusions on the efficacy of light therapy, it is being used to treat eating disorders, particularly in cases where antidepressants and established psychotherapies fail to be effective.

References

1. National Institute of Mental Health (NIMH). "Psychotherapies," October 2008.

2. Sholt, Michal and Gavron, Tami. "Therapeutic Qualities of Clay-work in Art Therapy and Psychotherapy: A Review" Journal of the American Art Therapy Association, 2006.

3. Eating Disorder Hope. "Eating Disorder Treatment," November 2015.

4. Wilson, George F. and Philips, Kelley L. "Concepts and Definitions Used in Quality Assurance and Utilization Review" *Manual of Psychiatric Quality Assurance*, American Psychiatric Association, 2005.

Chapter 42

Pharmacotherapy: Medications For Eating Disorders

Pharmacotherapy

Although medication alone cannot cure eating disorders, pharmacotherapy often plays a role in the treatment and recovery process. When used along with psychotherapy and nutritional guidance, medications such as antidepressants can help patients with eating disorders stabilize their mental and physical condition and control their symptoms. Prescription drugs may help people with bulimia suppress their urges to binge and purge, for instance, and may help people with anorexia manage their obsessive thinking about food and weight. A medication that benefits one patient might not work effectively for another, however, so it is important to consider different options. In addition, all medications involve side effects, so patients must weigh the risks of each drug against its possible health benefits.

There are three main categories of medications that are commonly used in the treatment of eating disorders:

- medications to restore body chemistry and manage the physical damage done by severe caloric restriction or repeated bingeing and purging episodes;

- medications to treat physical and mental health conditions that frequently co-exist with eating disorders and complicate treatment;

- psychiatric medications to treat the underlying depression, anxiety, obsessive-compulsive disorder, and other mental health conditions that often affect people with eating disorders.

"Pharmacotherapy: Medications For Eating Disorders," © 2017 Omnigraphics. Reviewed March 2017.

Medications To Manage Physical Damage

A variety of physical and mental health conditions often coexist with eating disorders and complicate the treatment process. Many people with eating disorders also have clinical psychiatric disorders such as depression, anxiety, bipolar, obsessive-compulsive, attention deficit, and posttraumatic stress. Medications are available to help patients manage the symptoms of these conditions in order to improve their ability to recover from eating disorders. Physical health conditions such as diabetes and celiac disease may also coexist with eating disorders. The special nutritional requirements associated with these conditions may impede the treatment of eating disorders. Medication can help patients manage their symptoms and eat a normal diet.

Medications To Address Coexisting Conditions

A variety of physical and mental health conditions often coexist with eating disorders and complicate the treatment process. Many people with eating disorders also have clinical psychiatric disorders such as depression, anxiety, bipolar, obsessive-compulsive, attention deficit, and posttraumatic stress. Medications are available to help patients manage the symptoms of these conditions in order to improve their ability to recover from eating disorders. Physical health conditions such as diabetes and celiac disease may also coexist with eating disorders. The special nutritional requirements associated with these conditions may impede the treatment of eating disorders. Medication can help patients manage their symptoms and eat a normal diet.

Psychiatric Medications For Eating Disorders

Antidepressants, mood stabilizers, and other psychiatric medications are often prescribed to treat eating disorders. Eating disorders are considered a form of psychiatric illness, and many people with eating disorders also have symptoms of depression, anxiety, and other psychiatric conditions. The most common types of psychiatric medications used in the treatment of eating disorders include:

- **Selective serotonin reuptake inhibitors (SSRI)**

  This category of antidepressant drugs works by increasing the level of serotonin (a chemical that affects mood) in the brain. SSRIs are commonly used to treat depression, anxiety, and obsessive-compulsive disorder. Fluoxetine (Prozac) is the only medication approved by the U.S. Food and Drug Administration (FDA) for the treatment of bulimia. Research suggests that fluoxetine may also help people with anorexia overcome underlying depression and maintain a healthy weight once they have brought their eating under control. Other commonly prescribed SSRIs include sertraline (Zoloft), fluvoxamine (Luvox), citalopram (Celexa), and paroxetine (Paxil). Although SSRIs well-tolerated by most people, some experience such side effects as drowsiness, weight gain, agitation, and loss of interest in sex.

- **Tricyclic antidepressants (TCAs) and monoamine oxidase inhibitors (MAOIs)**

These categories of antidepressant drugs have long been used to treat depression, panic disorder, and chronic pain. There is also some evidence that they may be effective in treating eating disorders, especially bulimia. They have more side effects than SSRIs, however, including dry mouth, headaches, blurred vision, dizziness, nausea, drowsiness, and insomnia. Examples include imipramine (Tofranil) and despiramine (Norpramin).

- **Other antidepressants**

Other types of antidepressants that are not related to SSRIs, TCAs, and MAOIs are also prescribed in the treatment of eating disorders. Medications like bupropion (Wellbutrin) and trazodone (Desyrel) work by increasing the levels of certain neurotransmitters, like norepinephrine, serotonin, and dopamine.

- **Mood stabilizers**

Mood stabilizers, such as lithium, are typically used in treating manic-depressive and bipolar disorders. Some research has indicated that they may also be helpful for patients with bulimia. Since these medications may cause weight loss, however, they are not usually considered for patients with anorexia.

- **Antipsychotics**

Olanzapine (Zyprexa) is an antipsychotic drug that is often prescribed for schizophrenia. Research has shown that it can also help some anorexia patients gain weight and overcome their obsessive thinking about food. Although many people tolerate olanzapine well, there is a risk of lightheadedness, dizziness, drowsiness, weakness, and tardive dyskinesia (a movement disorder).

- **Anticonvulsants**

The anti-seizure medication topiramate (Topamax) has been shown to help some people with bulimia suppress their urge to binge and purge and reduce their preoccupation with eating and weight. It can involve side effects, however, such as nausea, constipation or diarrhea, dizziness, drowsiness, insomnia, loss of appetite, and weight loss.

- **Central nervous system stimulants**

  Lisdexamfetamine dimesylate (Vyvanse), a medication that was developed to treat attention deficit hyperactivity disorder (ADHD), received FDA approval for the treatment of binge eating disorder in 2015. It has been shown to help adults who compulsively overeat to manage their urge to binge. However, Vyvanse is not approved as a medication to promote weight loss.

Vyvanse To Treat Binge Eating Disorder

The U.S. Food and Drug Administration (FDA) expanded the approved uses of Vyvanse (lisdexamfetamine dimesylate) to treat binge eating disorder in adults. The drug is the first FDA-approved medication to treat this condition.

In binge eating disorder, patients have recurrent episodes of compulsive overeating during which they consume larger amounts of food than normal and experience the sense that they lack control. Patients with this condition eat when they are not hungry and often eat to the point of being uncomfortably full. Patients may feel ashamed and embarrassed by how much they are eating, which can result in social isolation. Binge eating disorder may lead to weight gain and to health problems related to obesity.

"Binge eating can cause serious health problems and difficulties with work, home, and social life," said Mitchell Mathis, M.D., director of the Division of Psychiatry Products in the FDA's Center for Drug Evaluation and Research. "The approval of Vyvanse provides physicians and patients with an effective option to help curb episodes of binge eating."

Vyvanse was reviewed under the FDA's priority review program, which provides for an expedited review of drugs that are intended to treat a serious disease or condition and may provide a significant improvement over available therapy.

The efficacy of Vyvanse in treating binge eating disorder was shown in two clinical studies that included 724 adults with moderate-to-severe binge eating disorder. In the studies, participants taking Vyvanse experienced a decrease in the number of binge eating days per week and had fewer obsessive-compulsive binge eating behaviors compared to those on the inactive pill (placebo).

Vyvanse is dispensed with a Medication Guide for patients, which provides important information about the medication's use and risks. The most serious risks include psychiatric problems and heart complications, including sudden death in people who have heart problems or heart defects, and stroke and heart attack in adults. Central nervous system stimulants, like Vyvanse, may cause psychotic or manic symptoms, such as hallucinations, delusional thinking, or mania, even in individuals without a prior history of psychotic illness.

(Source: "FDA Expands Uses Of Vyvanse To Treat Binge Eating Disorder," U.S. Food and Drug Administration (FDA).)

References

1. Marks, Hedy. "How Medication Treats Eating Disorders," Everyday Health, May 10, 2010.

2. "Medications/Drugs to Treat Eating Disorders," Eating Disorder Referral and Information Center, n.d.

3. Tracy, Natasha. "Medications for Eating Disorders," Healthy Place, January 10, 2012.

Chapter 43

Improving Your Body Image And Self-Esteem

How Can I Deal With Body Image Issues?

Everyone has something they would like to change about their bodies. But you'll be happier if you focus on the things you like about your body—and your whole self. Need some help? Check out some tips given below:

- **List your great traits.** If you start to criticize your body, tell yourself to stop. Instead, think about what you like about yourself, both inside and out.

- **Know your power.** Hey, your body is not just a place to hang your clothes! It can do some truly amazing things. Focus on how strong and healthy your body can be.

- **Treat your body well.** Eat right, sleep tight, and get moving. You'll look and feel your best—and you'll be pretty proud of yourself too.

- **Give your body a treat.** Take a nice bubble bath, do some stretching, or just curl up on a comfy couch. Do something soothing.

- **Mind your media.** Try not to let models and actresses affect how you think you should look. They get lots of help from makeup artists, personal trainers, and photo fixers. And advertisers often use a focus on thinness to get people to buy stuff. Don't let them mess with your mind!

About This Chapter: Text under the heading "How Can I Deal With Body Image Issues?" is excerpted from "Having Body Image Issues," GirlsHealth.gov, Office on Women's Health (OWH), January 7, 2015; Text under the heading "What Is Self-Esteem?" is excerpted from "Self-Esteem," U.S. Department of Veterans Affairs (VA), July 2013. Reviewed March 2017; Text under the heading "Ways To Build Self-Esteem" is excerpted from "Ways To Build Self-Esteem," GirlsHealth.gov, Office on Women's Health (OWH), February 16, 2011. Reviewed March 2017.

- **Let yourself shine.** A lot of how we look comes from how we carry ourselves. Feeling proud, walking tall, and smiling big can boost your beauty—and your mood.

- **Find fab friends.** Your best bet is to hang out with people who accept you for you! And work with your friends to support each other.

If you can't seem to accept how you look, talk to an adult you trust. You can get help feeling better about your body.

Learning To Love What You See In The Mirror

Parents' attitudes about appearance and diet can affect their kids' attitudes.

We all want to look our best, but a healthy body is not always linked to appearance. In fact, healthy bodies come in all shapes and sizes! Changing your body image means changing the way you think about your body. At the same time, healthy lifestyle choices are also key to improving body image.

- Healthy eating can promote healthy skin and hair, along with strong bones.

- Regular exercise has been shown to boost self-esteem, self-image, and energy levels.

- Plenty of rest is key to stress management.

(Source: "Body Image," Office on Women's Health (OWH), U.S. Department of Health and Human Services (HHS).)

What Is Self-Esteem?

- Self-esteem is a way of thinking, feeling, and acting that implies that you accept, respect, and believe in yourself.

- When you accept yourself, you are okay with both the good and not so good things about yourself.

- When you respect yourself, you treat yourself well in much the same way you would treat someone else you respect.

- To believe in yourself means that you feel you deserve to have the good things in life. It also means that you have confidence that you can make choices and take actions that will have a positive effect on your life.

- Part of self-esteem is knowing that you are important enough to take good care of yourself by making good choices for yourself. For example, choosing nutritious food for your body, exercising, giving yourself time to relax, etc.

- Self-esteem doesn't mean you think you are better or more important than other people are, it means that you respect and value yourself as much as other people.

- Self-esteem needs to come from within and not be dependent on external sources such as material possessions, your status, or approval from others.

- Having self-esteem also means you don't have to put other people down to feel good about yourself.

Rate Your Self-Esteem

If you have healthy self-esteem, you probably will agree with some or most of the following statements:

- I feel good about who I am.
- I am proud of what I can do, but don't need to show off.
- I know there are some things that I'm good at and some things I need to improve.
- I feel it is okay if I win or if I lose.
- I usually think, "I can do this," before I do something.
- I am eager to learn new things.
- I can handle criticism.
- I like to try to do things without help, but I don't mind asking for help if I need it.
- I like myself.

(Source: "Self-Esteem And Self-Confidence," Office on Women's Health (OWH), U.S. Department of Health and Human Services (HHS).)

Signs Of Low And High Self-Esteem

Signs Of Low Self-Esteem

- Lack of confidence

- Negative view of life

- Perfectionistic attitude

- Mistrusting others inappropriately

- Blaming behavior

- Fear of taking appropriate risks

- Feelings of being unloved and unlovable

- Dependence on others to make decisions

- Fear of being ridiculed

Signs Of High Self-Esteem

- Confidence

- Self-direction

- Non-blaming behavior

- Awareness of personal strengths

- Ability to make mistakes and learn from them

- Ability to accept mistakes from others

- Optimism

- Ability to solve problems

- Independent and cooperative attitude

- Feeling comfortable with a wide range of emotions

- Ability to appropriately trust others

- Good sense of personal limitations

- Ability to set boundaries and say no

- Good self-care

Causes Of Low Self-Esteem

Nobody is born with low self-esteem; it's something that is learned. It is the result of filtering opinions, comments, looks, suggestions, and actions of those around us through a person's own feelings and self-image.

Some possible early causes of low self-esteem:

- Overly critical parents (never good enough, feelings of inferiority or self-criticism)

- Significant childhood losses (abandonment, insecurity)

- Parental abuse, alcoholism, neglect, or rejection (unreliable family atmosphere resulting in lack of trust, insecurity, inadequacy or worthlessness, anger, guilt, denying feelings)

- Parental overprotectiveness (lack of confidence)

- Parental overindulgence (feelings of being cheated and insecure because life does not continue to provide what they learnt to expect as a child)

Some possible later contributors to low self-esteem:

- Negative or controlling personal relationships

- Negative experiences on the job

- Messages from society

Even if low self-esteem had its roots in childhood, you can learn to identify and challenge the assumptions you consciously or unconsciously have about yourself.

- Take notice of and become more consciously aware of your needs.

- Acknowledge the importance of self-nurturing and self-care activities and take appropriate steps in that direction.

- Recognize and take pride in your accomplishments.

- Focus on problem solving.

Ways To Build Self-Esteem

Having healthy or high self-esteem means that you feel good about yourself and are proud of what you can do. Having high self-esteem can help you to think positively, deal better with stress, and boost your drive to work hard. Having high self-esteem can also make it easier to try new things. Before you try something new, you think, "I can do this," and not, "This is too hard. I'll never be able to do this."

If you have an illness or disability, how does it affect your self-esteem? Do you find your self-esteem is affected by how you think others see you? Do people put you down or bully you? This can put your self-esteem at risk. If you need a self-esteem boost, take these steps:

- **Ask yourself what you are really good at and enjoy doing.** Everyone is good at something. When you're feeling bad about yourself, just think, "I'm good at art" (or computers or playing an instrument or whatever you're good at). You might make a list of your great traits and talents, too. And remember that it's okay not to be great at everything.

- **Push yourself to try new things.** If you try something new and fail, that's okay. Everyone fails sometime. Try to figure out what went wrong, so you can try again in a new way. Keep trying, and don't give up. In time, you'll figure out how to succeed.

- **Always give your best effort, and take pride in your effort.** When you accomplish a goal, celebrate over a family meal or treat yourself to a fun outing.

- **If you need help, ask for it.** Talking to a parent, teacher, or friend can help you come up with different ways to solve a problem. This is called brainstorming. Make a list of your possible solutions. Put the ones that you think will work the best at the top. Then rehearse them ahead of time so that you'll know exactly what you're going to do or say when the problem comes up. If your first plan doesn't work, then go on to Plan B. If Plan B doesn't work, go on to Plan C, and so on.

- **Join a support group.** Finding out how other kids deal with illnesses or disabilities can help you cope. Ask your doctor, teachers, or parents for help finding a support group in your community or online.

- **Volunteer to do something at school or in your community.** For instance, you could tutor a younger child or take care of the plants in the community center lobby. You might also volunteer to do some chores at home.

- **Look for ways to take more control over your life.** For instance, every student who has needs related to an illness or disability in school must have an Individualized Education Plan, or IEP. Your IEP describes your goals during the school year and any support that you'll need to help achieve those goals. Get involved with the development of your IEP. Attend any IEP meetings. Tell your parents, teachers, and others involved in your IEP what you think your goals at school should be and what would help you achieve them. It's your education, and you get a say in what happens!

- **Speak up for yourself.** This can be difficult if you're shy. But it can get easier with practice. Learn to communicate your needs and don't hesitate to ask for something.

- **Work on trying to feel good about how you look.** Everyone has some things they like and don't like about their bodies. It pays to focus on the positives since your body image, or how you feel about your looks, can affect your self-esteem. And remember that real beauty comes from the inside! If you like makeup and clothes, ask for help dealing with any obstacles your illness or disability might present.

- **If you still find that you are not feeling good about yourself, talk to your parents, a school counselor, or your doctor because you may be at risk for depression.** You can also ask the school nurse if your school offers counseling for help through tough times.

Part Five
Maintaining Healthy Eating And Fitness Habits

Chapter 44

Building A Healthy Eating Style

The Importance Of Healthy Eating

Dietary Guidelines Advisory Committee (DGAC) 2015 Overarching Themes:

- **The Problem.** More than two-thirds of adults and nearly one-third of children and youth are overweight or obese, further exacerbating poor health profiles and increasing risks for chronic diseases and their co-morbidities. High chronic disease rates and elevated population disease risk profiles have persisted for more than two decades and disproportionately affect low-income and underserved communities. These diseases focus the attention of the U.S. healthcare system on disease treatment rather than prevention; increase already strained healthcare costs; and reduce overall population health, quality of life, and national productivity. Other less common, but important, diet- and lifestyle-related health problems, including poor bone health and certain neuropsychological disorders and congenital anomalies, pose further serious concerns.

- **The Gap.** The dietary patterns of the American public are suboptimal and are causally related to poor individual and population health and higher chronic disease rates. Few, if any, improvements in consumers' food choices have been seen in recent decades. On average, the U.S. diet is low in vegetables, fruits, and whole grains, and high in sodium, calories, saturated fat, refined grains, and added sugars. Underconsumption of

About This Chapter: About This Chapter: Text under the heading "The Importance Of Healthy Eating" is excerpted from "Scientific Report of the 2015 Dietary Guidelines Advisory Committee," Office of Disease Prevention and Health Promotion (ODPHP), U.S. Department of Health and Human Services (HHS), February 19, 2015; Text under the heading "How To Build A Healthy Eating Style?" is excerpted from "MyPlate," ChooseMyPlate.gov, U.S. Department of Agriculture (USDA), January 25, 2017.

the essential nutrients such as vitamin D, calcium, potassium, and fiber are public health concerns for the majority of the U.S. population, and iron intake is of concern among adolescents and premenopausal females. Health disparities exist in population access to affordable healthy foods. Eating behaviors of individuals are shaped by complex but modifiable factors, including individual, personal, household, social/cultural, community/environmental, systems/sectorial and policy-level factors. However, a dynamic and rapidly evolving food environment epitomized by the abundance of highly processed, convenient, lower-cost, energy-dense, nutrient-poor foods makes it particularly challenging to implement health promoting diet-related behavior changes at individual and population levels.

- **The Dietary Patterns.** Current research provides evidence of moderate to strong links between healthy dietary patterns, lower risks of obesity and chronic diseases, particularly cardiovascular disease, hypertension, type 2 diabetes and certain cancers. Emerging evidence also suggests that relationships may exist between dietary patterns and some neurocognitive disorders and congenital anomalies. **The overall body of evidence examined by the 2015 DGAC identifies that a healthy dietary pattern is higher in vegetables, fruits, whole grains, low- or non-fat dairy, seafood, legumes, and nuts; moderate in alcohol (among adults); lower in red and processed meats; and low in sugar-sweetened foods and drinks and refined grains.** Additional strong evidence shows that it is not necessary to eliminate food groups or conform to a single dietary pattern to achieve healthy dietary patterns. Rather, individuals can combine foods in a variety of flexible ways to achieve healthy dietary patterns, and these strategies should be tailored to meet the individual's health needs, dietary preferences and cultural traditions. Current research also strongly demonstrates that regular physical activity promotes health and reduces chronic disease risk.

In summary, the research base reviewed by the 2015 DGAC provides clear and consistent evidence that persistent, prevalent, preventable health problems, notably overweight and obesity, cardiovascular diseases, diabetes, and certain cancers, have severely and adversely affected the health of the U.S. population across all stages of the lifespan for decades and raise the urgency for immediate attention and bold action. Evidence points to specific areas of food and nutrient concern in the current U.S. diet. Moderate to strong evidence pinpoints the characteristics of healthy dietary and physical activity patterns established to reduce chronic disease risk, prevent and better manage overweight and obesity, and promote health and well-being across the lifespan.

How To Build A Healthy Eating Style?

MyPlate is a reminder to find your healthy eating style and build it throughout your lifetime. Everything you eat and drink matters. The right mix can help you be healthier now and in the future. This means:

- Focus on variety, amount, and nutrition.

- Choose foods and beverages with less saturated fat, sodium, and added sugars.

- Start with small changes to build healthier eating styles.

- Support healthy eating for everyone.

Eating healthy is a journey shaped by many factors, including our stage of life, situations, preferences, access to food, culture, traditions, and the personal decisions we make over time. All your food and beverage choices count. MyPlate offers ideas and tips to help you create a healthier eating style that meets your individual needs and improves your health.

Build A Healthy Eating Style

All food and beverage choices matter—focus on variety, amount, and nutrition.

- Focus on making healthy food and beverage choices from all five food groups including fruits, vegetables, grains, protein foods, and dairy to get the nutrients you need.

- Eat the right amount of calories for you based on your age, sex, height, weight, and physical activity level.

- Building a healthier eating style can help you avoid overweight and obesity and reduce your risk of diseases such as heart disease, diabetes, and cancer.

Choose an eating style low in saturated fat, sodium, and added sugars.

- Use Nutrition Facts Labels and ingredient lists to find amounts of saturated fat, sodium, and added sugars in the foods and beverages you choose.

- Look for food and drink choices that are lower in saturated fat, sodium, and added sugar.

- Eating fewer calories from foods high in saturated fat and added sugars can help you manage your calories and prevent overweight and obesity. Most of us eat too many foods that are high in saturated fat and added sugar.

- Eating foods with less sodium can reduce your risk of high blood pressure.

Make small changes to create a healthier eating style.

- Think of each change as a personal "win" on your path to living healthier. Each MyWin is a change you make to build your healthy eating style. Find little victories that fit into your lifestyle and celebrate as a MyWin!

- Start with a few of these small changes.

- Make half your plate fruits and vegetables.

- Focus on whole fruits.

- Vary your veggies.

- Make half your grains whole grains.

- Move to low-fat and fat-free dairy.

- Vary your protein routine.

- Eat and drink the right amount for you.

Support healthy eating for everyone.

- Create settings where healthy choices are available and affordable to you and others in your community.

- Professionals, policymakers, partners, industry, families, and individuals can help others in their journey to make healthy eating a part of their lives.

Chapter 45
What Should You Really Eat?

Importance Of Healthy Diet

Eating healthy means getting enough vitamins, minerals, and other nutrients—and limiting unhealthy foods and drinks. Eating healthy also means getting the number of calories that's right for you (not eating too much or too little).

To eat healthy, be sure to get plenty of:

- Vegetables, fruits, whole grains, and fat-free or low-fat dairy products

- Seafood, lean meats and poultry, eggs, beans, peas, seeds, and nuts

It's also important to limit:

- Sodium (salt)

- Added sugars—like refined (regular) sugar, brown sugar, corn syrup, high-fructose corn syrup, and honey

- Saturated fats, which come from animal products like cheese, fatty meats, whole milk, and butter, and plant products like palm and coconut oils

- *Trans* fats, which may be in foods like stick margarines, coffee creamers, and some desserts

- Refined grains which are in foods like cookies, white bread, and some snack foods

About This Chapter: This chapter includes text excerpted from "Eat Healthy," Office of Disease Prevention and Health Promotion (ODPHP), U.S. Department of Health and Human Services (HHS), January 26, 2017.

A Healthy Diet Can Help Keep You Healthy

Eating healthy is good for your overall health. Making smart food choices can also help you manage your weight and lower your risk for certain chronic (long-term) diseases.

The Guidelines

- **Follow a healthy eating pattern across the lifespan.** All food and beverage choices matter. Choose a healthy eating pattern at an appropriate calorie level to help achieve and maintain a healthy body weight, support nutrient adequacy, and reduce the risk of chronic disease.

- **Focus on variety, nutrient density, and amount.** To meet nutrient needs within calorie limits, choose a variety of nutrient-dense foods across and within all food groups in recommended amounts.

- **Limit calories from added sugars and saturated fats and reduce sodium intake.** Consume an eating pattern low in added sugars, saturated fats, and sodium. Cut back on foods and beverages higher in these components to amounts that fit within healthy eating patterns.

- **Shift to healthier food and beverage choices.** Choose nutrient-dense foods and beverages across and within all food groups in place of less healthy choices. Consider cultural and personal preferences to make these shifts easier to accomplish and maintain.

- **Support healthy eating patterns for all.** Everyone has a role in helping to create and support healthy eating patterns in multiple settings nationwide, from home to school to work to communities.

(Source: "Key Elements Of Healthy Eating Patterns," U.S. Department of Health and Human Services (HHS).)

When you eat healthy foods—and limit unhealthy foods—you can reduce your risk for:

- Heart disease

- Type 2 diabetes

- High blood pressure

- Some types of cancer

- Osteoporosis (bone loss)

What You Need To Do

Making small changes to your eating habits can make a big difference for your health over time. Here are some tips and tools you can use to get started.

Keep A Food Diary

Knowing what you eat now will help you figure out what you want to change.

- When you eat
- What and how much you eat
- Where you are and who you are with when you eat
- How you are feeling when you eat

Shop Smart At The Grocery Store

The next time you go food shopping:

- Make a shopping list ahead of time. Only buy what's on your list.
- Don't shop while you are hungry—eat something before you go to the store.

Use these tips to buy healthy foods:

- Try a variety of vegetables and fruits in different colors.
- Look for low-sodium foods from this list.
- Choose fat-free or low-fat dairy products.
- Replace old favorites with options that have fewer calories and less saturated fat.
- Choose foods with whole grains—like 100 percent whole-wheat or whole-grain bread, cereal, and pasta.
- Buy lean cuts of meat and poultry and other foods with protein—like fish, seafood, and beans.
- Save money by getting fruits and vegetables in season or on sale.

Read The Nutrition Facts Label

Understanding the Nutrition Facts Label on food packages can help you make healthy choices.

First, look at the serving size and the number of servings per package—there may be more than 1 serving!

Next, check out the percent Daily Value (%DV) column. The DV lets you know if a food is higher or lower in certain nutrients. Look for foods that are:

- Lower in sodium and saturated fat (5 percent DV or less)

- Higher in fiber, calcium, potassium, and vitamin D (20 percent DV or more)

Read the ingredients list, too. To limit added sugars in your food, make sure that added sugars are not listed in the first few ingredients. Names for added sugars include: sugar, corn syrup, high-fructose corn syrup, fruit juice concentrate, maltose, dextrose, sucrose, honey, and maple syrup.

Be A Healthy Family

Parents and caregivers are important role models for healthy eating. You can teach kids how to choose and prepare healthy foods.

- Take your child with you to the store and explain the choices you make.

- Turn cooking into a fun activity for the whole family.

Eat Healthy Away From Home

You can make smart food choices wherever you are—at work, in your favorite restaurant, or out running errands. Try these tips for eating healthy even when you are away from home:

- At lunch, have a sandwich on whole-grain bread instead of white bread.

- Skip the soda—drink water instead.

- In a restaurant, choose dishes that are steamed, baked, or grilled instead of fried.

- On a long drive or shopping trip, pack healthy snacks like fruit, unsalted nuts, or low-fat string cheese sticks.

If You Are Worried About Your Eating Habits, Talk To A Doctor

If you need help making healthier food choices, your doctor or a registered dietitian can help. A registered dietitian is a health professional who helps people with healthy eating.

If you make an appointment to talk about your eating habits, be sure to take a food diary with you to help start the conversation.

About half of all American adults—117 million individuals—have one or more preventable chronic diseases, many of which are related to poor quality eating patterns and physical inactivity. These include cardiovascular disease, high blood pressure, type 2 diabetes, some cancers, and poor bone health. More than two-thirds of adults and nearly one-third of children and youth are overweight or obese.

(Source: "Nutrition And Health Are Closely Related," U.S. Department of Health and Human Services (HHS).)

Chapter 46
Improving Your Eating Habits

When it comes to eating, we have strong habits. Some are good ("I always eat breakfast"), and some are not so good ("I always clean my plate"). Although many of our eating habits were established during childhood, it doesn't mean it's too late to change them.

Making sudden, radical changes to eating habits such as eating nothing but cabbage soup, can lead to short-term weight loss. However, such radical changes are neither healthy nor a good idea, and won't be successful in the long run. Permanently improving your eating habits requires a thoughtful approach in which you Reflect, Replace, and Reinforce.

- **REFLECT** on all of your specific eating habits, both bad and good; and, your common triggers for unhealthy eating.

- **REPLACE** your unhealthy eating habits with healthier ones.

- **REINFORCE** your new, healthier eating habits.

Reflect, Replace, Reinforce: A Process For Improving Your Eating Habits

- **Create a list of your eating habits.** Keeping a food diary for a few days, in which you write down everything you eat and the time of day you ate it, will help you uncover your habits. For example, you might discover that you always seek a sweet snack to get you through the mid-afternoon energy slump. It's good to note how you were feeling when you decided to eat, especially if you were eating when not hungry. Were you tired? Stressed out?

About This Chapter: This chapter includes text excerpted from "Improving Your Eating Habits," Centers for Disease Control and Prevention (CDC), May 15, 2015.

- **Highlight the habits** on your list that may be leading you to overeat. Common eating habits that can lead to weight gain are:

  - Eating too fast

  - Always cleaning your plate

  - Eating when not hungry

  - Eating while standing up (may lead to eating mindlessly or too quickly)

  - Always eating dessert

  - Skipping meals (or maybe just breakfast)

- **Look at the unhealthy eating habits** you've highlighted. Be sure you've identified all the triggers that cause you to engage in those habits. Identify a few you'd like to work on improving first. Don't forget to pat yourself on the back for the things you're doing right. Maybe you almost always eat fruit for dessert, or you drink low-fat or fat-free milk. These are good habits! Recognizing your successes will help encourage you to make more changes.

- **Create a list of "cues"** by reviewing your food diary to become more aware of when and where you're "triggered" to eat for reasons other than hunger. Note how you are typically feeling at those times. Often an environmental "cue," or a particular emotional state, is what encourages eating for non-hunger reasons.

- **Identify triggers.** Common triggers for eating when not hungry are:

  - Opening up the cabinet and seeing your favorite snack food.

  - Sitting at home watching television.

  - Before or after a stressful meeting or situation at work.

  - Coming home after work and having no idea what's for dinner.

  - Having someone offer you a dish they made "just for you!"

  - Walking past a candy dish on the counter.

  - Sitting in the break room beside the vending machine.

  - Seeing a plate of doughnuts at the morning staff meeting.

  - Swinging through your favorite drive-through every morning.

  - Feeling bored or tired and thinking food might offer a pick-me-up.

- **Circle the "cues" on your list that you face on a daily or weekly basis.** Going home for the Thanksgiving holiday may be a trigger for you to overeat, and eventually, you want to have a plan for as many eating cues as you can. But for now, focus on the ones you face more often.

- **Ask yourself** these questions for each "cue" you've circled:

- **Is there anything I can do to avoid the cue or situation?** This option works best for cues that don't involve others. For example, could you choose a different route to work to avoid stopping at a fast food restaurant on the way? Is there another place in the break room where you can sit so you're not next to the vending machine?

- **For things I can't avoid, can I do something differently that would be healthier?** Obviously, you can't avoid all situations that trigger your unhealthy eating habits, like staff meetings at work. In these situations, evaluate your options. Could you suggest or bring healthier snacks or beverages? Could you offer to take notes to distract your attention? Could you sit farther away from the food so it won't be as easy to grab something? Could you plan ahead and eat a healthy snack before the meeting?

- **Replace unhealthy habits with new, healthy ones.** For example, in reflecting upon your eating habits, you may realize that you eat too fast when you eat alone. So, make a commitment to share a lunch each week with a colleague, or have a neighbor over for dinner one night a week. Other strategies might include putting your fork down between bites or minimizing other distractions (i.e., watching the news during dinner) that might keep you from paying attention to how quickly—and how much—you're eating.

Here are more ideas to help you replace unhealthy habits:

- **Eat more slowly.** If you eat too quickly, you may "clean your plate" instead of paying attention to whether your hunger is satisfied.

- **Eat only when you're truly hungry** instead of when you are tired, anxious, or feeling an emotion besides hunger. If you find yourself eating when you are experiencing an emotion besides hunger, such as boredom or anxiety, try to find a non-eating activity to do instead. You may find a quick walk or phone call with a friend helps you feel better.

- **Plan meals ahead of time** to ensure that you eat a healthy well-balanced meal.

- **Reinforce your new, healthy habits and be patient with yourself.** Habits take time to develop. It doesn't happen overnight. When you do find yourself engaging in an unhealthy habit, stop as quickly as possible and ask yourself:

- Why do I do this?

- When did I start doing this?

- What changes do I need to make?

Be careful not to berate yourself or think that one mistake "blows" a whole day's worth of healthy habits. You can do it! It just takes one day at a time!

Chapter 47

Healthy Eating And Weight Management

Eat Healthfully And Enjoy It!

A healthy eating plan that helps you manage your weight includes a variety of foods you may not have considered. If "healthy eating" makes you think about the foods you can't have, try refocusing on all the new foods you can eat:

- **Fresh, Frozen, or Canned Fruits**—don't think just apples or bananas. All fresh, frozen, or canned fruits are great choices. Be sure to try some "exotic" fruits, too. How about a mango? Or a juicy pineapple or kiwi fruit! When your favorite fresh fruits aren't in season, try a frozen, canned, or dried variety of a fresh fruit you enjoy. One caution about canned fruits is that they may contain added sugars or syrups. Be sure and choose canned varieties of fruit packed in water or in their own juice.

- **Fresh, Frozen, or Canned Vegetables**—try something new. You may find that you love grilled vegetables or steamed vegetables with an herb you haven't tried like rosemary. You can sauté (panfry) vegetables in a non-stick pan with a small amount of cooking spray. Or try frozen or canned vegetables for a quick side dish—just microwave and serve. When trying canned vegetables, look for vegetables without added salt, butter, or

About This Chapter: Text beginning with the heading "Eat Healthfully And Enjoy It!" is excerpted from "Healthy Eating For A Healthy Weight," Centers for Disease Control and Prevention (CDC), September 8, 2016; Text beginning with the heading "If I Cut Calories, Won't I Be Hungry?" is excerpted from "Eat More, Weigh Less?" Centers for Disease Control and Prevention (CDC), May 15, 2015; Text beginning with the heading "Advantages Of A Healthy Eating Plan" is excerpted from "Aim For A Healthy Weight," National Heart, Lung, and Blood Institute (NHLBI), February 13, 2013. Reviewed March 2017; Text beginning with the heading "Weight Management" is excerpted from "Weight Management," Federal Occupational Health (FOH), U.S. Department of Health and Human Services (HHS), February 15, 2013. Reviewed March 2017.

cream sauces. Commit to going to the produce department and trying a new vegetable each week.

- **Calcium-rich foods**—you may automatically think of a glass of low-fat or fat-free milk when someone says "eat more dairy products." But what about low-fat and fat-free yogurts without added sugars? These come in a wide variety of flavors and can be a great dessert substitute for those with a sweet tooth.

- **A new twist on an old favorite**—if your favorite recipe calls for frying fish or breaded chicken, try healthier variations using baking or grilling. Maybe even try a recipe that uses dry beans in place of higher-fat meats. Ask around or search the Internet and magazines for recipes with fewer calories—you might be surprised to find you have a new favorite dish!

Do I Have To Give Up My Favorite Comfort Food?

No! Healthy eating is all about balance. You can enjoy your favorite foods even if they are high in calories, fat or added sugars. The key is eating them only once in awhile, and balancing them out with healthier foods and more physical activity.

Some general tips for comfort foods:

- **Eat them less often.** If you normally eat these foods every day, cut back to once a week or once a month. You'll be cutting your calories because you're not having the food as often.

- **Eat smaller amounts.** If your favorite higher-calorie food is a chocolate bar, have a smaller size or only half a bar.

- **Try a lower-calorie version.** Use lower-calorie ingredients or prepare food differently. For example, if your macaroni and cheese recipe uses whole milk, butter, and full-fat cheese, try remaking it with non-fat milk, less butter, light cream cheese, fresh spinach and tomatoes. Just remember to not increase your portion size.

If I Cut Calories, Won't I Be Hungry?

Research shows that people get full by the amount of food they eat, not the number of calories they take in. You can cut calories in your favorite foods by lowering the amount of fat and or increasing the amount of fiber-rich ingredients, such as vegetables or fruit.

Let's take macaroni and cheese as an example. The original recipe uses whole milk, butter, and full-fat cheese. This recipe has about 540 calories in one serving (1 cup).

Here's how to remake this recipe with fewer calories and less fat:

- Use 2 cups non-fat milk instead of 2 cups whole milk.

- Use 8 ounces light cream cheese instead of 2¼ cups full-fat cheddar cheese.

- Use 1 tablespoon butter instead of 2 or use 2 tablespoons of soft trans-fat free margarine.

- Add about 2 cups of fresh spinach and 1 cup diced tomatoes (or any other veggie you like).

Your redesigned mac and cheese now has 315 calories in one serving (1 cup). You can eat the same amount of mac and cheese with 225 fewer calories.

What Foods Will Fill Me Up?

To be able to cut calories without eating less and feeling hungry, you need to replace some higher calorie foods with foods that are lower in calories and fat and will fill you up. In general, this means foods with lots of water and fiber in them. The table below will help you make smart food choices that are part of a healthy eating plan.

Table 47.1. Smart Food Choices

These Foods Will Fill You Up With Less Calories. Choose Them *More* Often...	These Foods Can Pack More Calories Into Each Bite. Choose Them *Less* Often...
Fruits and Vegetables (prepared without added fat)	**Fried foods**
Spinach, broccoli, tomato, carrots, watermelon, berries, apples	Eggs fried in butter, fried vegetables, French fries
Low-fat and fat-free milk products	**Full-fat milk products**
Low- or fat-free milk, low or fat-free yogurt, low- or fat-free cottage cheese	Full-fat cheese, full-fat ice cream, whole and 2 percent milk
Broth-based soup	**Dry snack foods**
Vegetable-based soups, soups with chicken or beef broth, tomato soups (without cream)	Crackers or pretzels, cookies, chips, dried fruits
Whole grains	**Higher-fat and higher-sugar foods**
Brown rice, whole wheat bread, whole wheat pastas, popcorn	Croissants, margarine, shortening and butter, doughnuts, candy bars, cakes and pastries

Table 47.1. Continued

These Foods Will Fill You Up With Less Calories. Choose Them *More* Often...	These Foods Can Pack More Calories Into Each Bite. Choose Them *Less* Often...
Lean meat, poultry and fish	**Fatty cuts of meat**
Grilled salmon, chicken breast without skin, ground beef (lean or extra lean)	Bacon, brisket, ground beef (regular)
Legumes (beans and peas)	
Black, red kidney and pinto beans (without added fat), green peas, black-eyed peas	

Advantages Of A Healthy Eating Plan

A healthy eating plan gives your body the nutrients it needs every day while staying within your daily calorie goal for weight loss. A healthy eating plan also will lower your risk for heart disease and other health conditions.

A healthy eating plan:

- Emphasizes vegetables, fruits, whole grains, and fat-free or low-fat dairy products

- Includes lean meats, poultry, fish, beans, eggs, and nuts

- Limits saturated and trans fats, sodium, and added sugars

- Controls portion sizes

Calories

To lose weight, most people need to reduce the number of calories they get from food and beverages (energy IN) and increase their physical activity (energy OUT).

For a weight loss of 1–1 ½ pounds per week, daily intake should be reduced by 500 to 750 calories. In general:

- Eating plans that contain 1,200–1,500 calories each day will help most women lose weight safely.

- Eating plans that contain 1,500–1,800 calories each day are suitable for men and for women who weigh more or who exercise regularly.

Very low calorie diets of fewer than 800 calories per day should not be used unless you are being monitored by your doctor.

> ## Technically Speaking...
>
> The number of calories in a particular amount or weight of food is called "calorie density" or "energy density." Low-calorie-dense foods are ones that don't pack a lot of calories into each bite.
>
> Foods that have a lot of water or fiber and little fat are usually low in calorie density. They will help you feel full without an unnecessary amount of calories.

Tips For Eating Right

Small steps can help your family get on the road to maintaining a healthy weight. Choose a different tip each week for you and your family to try. See if you or they can add to the list. Here are a few:

Change Your Shopping Habits

- Eat before grocery shopping
- Make a grocery list before you shop
- Choose a checkout line without a candy display
- Buy and try serving a new fruit or vegetable (ever had jicama, fava beans, plantain, bok choy, star fruit, or papaya?)

Watch Your Portion Size

- Share an entree with someone
- If entrees are large, choose an appetizer or side dish
- Don't serve seconds
- Share dessert, or choose fruit instead
- Eat sweet foods in small amounts. To reduce temptation, don't keep sweets at home
- Cut or share high-calorie foods like cheese and chocolate into small pieces and only eat a few pieces
- Eat off smaller plates
- Skip buffets

Change The Way You Prepare Food

- Cut back on added fats and/or oils in cooking or spreads

- Grill, steam, or bake instead of frying

- Make foods flavorful with herbs, spices, and low-fat seasonings

- Use fat-free or low-fat sour cream, mayo, sauces, dressings, and condiments

- Serve several whole-grain foods every day

- Top off cereal with sliced apples or bananas

Change Your Eating Habits

- Keep to a regular eating schedule

- Eat together as a family most days of the week

- Eat before you get too hungry

- Make sure every family member eats breakfast every day

- Drink water before a meal

- Stop eating when you're full

- Don't eat late at night

- Try a green salad instead of fries

- Ask for salad dressing "on the side"

- Chew slowly every time you eat and remind others to enjoy every bite

- Serve water or low-fat milk at meals, instead of soda or other sugary drinks

- Pay attention to flavors and textures

- Instead of eating out, bring a healthy, low-calorie lunch to work and pack a healthy "brown bag" for your kids

- Provide fruits and vegetables for snacks

- Ask your sweetie to bring you fruit or flowers instead of chocolate

Weight Management

Lower your risk of developing serious health problems by maintaining a healthy weight—or safely lowering your weight, if you are overweight.

Maintain A Healthy Weight

Being overweight or obese can raise your risk of developing potentially serious health problems. However, maintaining a healthy weight is often as simple as eating right and getting regular physical activity. Maintaining or losing weight is formulaic:

- To maintain your weight, you need to burn as many calories as you take in

- To lose weight, you need to use more calories than you take in

Assess Your Weight

To find out where you stand, use the BMI calculator on this page. If you are overweight (your BMI is 25 or higher), combining a low-calorie, well-balanced diet with regular physical activity can help you let go of the extra weight.

Lose Weight

If you find from your BMI that you need to lose weight, remember that healthy weight loss isn't just about a "diet" or "program." The key to success is ongoing lifestyle choices that include long-term changes in daily eating and physical activity habits. Realistic goals with small and consistent wins will bring you back to a weight that is healthy for you.

Get A Daily Dose Of Physical Activity

- Everyone is different, but 30 minutes per day of moderate-intensity activities like brisk walking is a good start for most of us.

- Being physically active has the added benefit of burning calories, which can help with maintaining a healthy weight.

- It adds up! You don't have to do it all in one stretch—ten minutes here, 20 minutes there works well, too.

Healthy Eating For Weight Management

Low-And No-Calorie Alternatives

Sometimes all that's needed to lose weight are small adjustments—for instance, making the low-calorie choice of an apple versus a bag of chips for a snack—or making the no-calorie choice of tea or coffee instead of a soda.

Green Light Choices

Some foods, like the alternatives mentioned above, give you a nutritional "green light" like:

Fruits And Vegetables

Fruits and vegetables are a natural choice for nutritionally dense foods, so you can be generous in serving up these highly nourishing treats. In fact, according to ChooseMyPlate.gov, fruits and vegetables should make up half of your plate at any given meal—about 30 percent vegetables and 20 percent fruit. Choosing fruits and vegetables of different colors also adds variety in terms of flavor and nutrition.

How many servings of fruits and vegetables do you need each day? This depends on your age, sex, and levels of physical activity.

Whole Grain Foods

Grains should also account for a sizable portion of your plate—about 30 percent. The USDA recommends that whole grains make up at least half of those grains. Whole grains not only can give you more fiber, which helps you feel more satisfied.

Lean Sources Of Protein

Lean protein is important to a smart eating plan—it should make about 20 percent of your plate. There are many good sources of lean protein, including:

Dairy And Other Calcium-Rich Foods

Dairy products can be a good source of protein and calcium, but low-fat and no-fat dairy products are the most nutritionally dense. Other calcium-fortified food sources include cereals, breads, and some juices, as well as soy, rice, and nut beverages. Dark leafy vegetables, like turnip greens, kale, Chinese cabbage, and mustard greens, are additional sources of calcium.

Stay Hydrated

Drink low- and no-calorie beverages such as water, unsweetened tea and coffee, or flavored sparkling water. Foods like raw fruits and vegetables can also help keep you hydrated. Your body can have trouble distinguishing hunger from thirst pangs, so being well hydrated can often keep you from eating too much.

"Red Light" And "Yellow Light" Choices

While some foods clearly get the "green light" nutritionally, others deserve a yellow or even a red light. Fats, oils, sugars, and other high-calorie/low nutrition foods, should be approached with caution. Alcohol also gives you high calories with minimal nutrition, so if you're watching your calories and you want every calorie to count, avoid the empty calories in alcohol.

Portion Size

Watching your portion sizes is also important for losing or maintaining your ideal weight. Smaller portions mean fewer calories, and moderate-sized portions can help you maintain your weight. You can still have things you enjoy, just less of it. Have a "sliver," a "taste," a "bite," and savor the flavor.

Bottom Line

All most of us need to do is to make some adjustments—go for the low-or no-calorie choice and have more "green light" foods, avoiding red and yellow light foods. This can put you on the road to losing weight or maintaining your current healthy weight.

Chapter 48

Identifying The Right Weight For Your Height

"What's the right weight for my height?" is one of the most common questions girls and guys have. It seems like a simple question. But, for teens, it's not always an easy one to answer.

It's normal for two people who are the same height and age to have very different weights. First, not everyone goes through puberty at the same time: Some kids start developing as early as age 8 and others might not develop until age 14. Second, people have different body types. Some are more muscular or shaped differently than others.

You can't point to a number on a scale as the "right" number, but it is possible to find out if you are in a *healthy weight range* for your height and age. That's why doctors use body mass index (BMI).

People Grow And Develop Differently

Not everyone grows and develops on the same schedule, but most people go through a period of faster growth during their teens. During puberty, the body begins making hormones that spark physical changes like faster muscle growth (particularly in guys) and spurts in height. As the amount of muscle, fat, and bone in the body changes during this time, some people might gain weight more rapidly.

It can feel strange adjusting to a new body. But all that new weight gain can be perfectly fine—as long as body fat, muscle, and bone are in the right proportion.

About This Chapter: Text in this chapter is © 1995-2017. The Nemours Foundation/KidsHealth®. Reprinted with permission.

Figuring Out Fat Using BMI

Because weight is more complicated during our teens, doctors don't rely on weight alone to figure out if someone is in a healthy weight range. Instead, they use the body mass index, or BMI. BMI is a formula that doctors use to estimate how much body fat a person has based on his or her weight and height.

The BMI formula uses height and weight measurements to calculate a BMI number. This number is then plotted on a BMI chart, which helps tell a person whether he or she is in the underweight, healthy weight, overweight, or obese range.

The growth charts have lines for "percentiles." Like percentages, percentiles go from 0 to 100. The eight lines on the BMI growth charts show the 5th, 10th, 25th, 50th, 75th, 85th, 90th, and 95th percentiles. The 50th percentile line is the average BMI of the teens who were measured to make the chart.

When your BMI is plotted on the chart, the doctor can see how you compare with other people the same age and gender as you. Based on where your number is on the chart, a doctor will decide if your BMI is in the underweight, normal weight, overweight, or obese range.

There's a big range of normal on the chart: Anyone who falls between the 5th percentile and the 85th percentile is in the healthy weight range. If someone is at or above the 85th percentile line on the chart (but less than the 95th percentile), that person may be overweight. A BMI measurement over the 95th percentile line on the chart puts someone in the obese range.

What Does BMI Tell Us?

You can calculate BMI on your own, but it's a good idea to ask your doctor, school nurse, or other health professional to help you figure out what it means.

A doctor can use BMI results from past years to track whether you may be at risk for becoming overweight. Spotting this risk early on can be helpful because the person can then make changes in diet and exercise to help head off a weight problem.

BMI can be a good indicator of a person's body fat, but it doesn't always tell the full story. People can have a high BMI because they have a large frame or a lot of muscle (like a bodybuilder or athlete) instead of excess fat. Likewise, a small person with a small frame might have a normal BMI but could still have too much body fat. These are other good reasons to talk about your BMI with your doctor.

How Can I Be Sure I'm Not Overweight Or Underweight?

If you think you've gained too much weight or you're too skinny, a doctor can help you decide whether it's normal for you or whether you really have a weight problem. Your doctor has measured your height and weight and has plotted your BMI over time. So he or she can tell whether you're growing normally.

If your doctor is concerned about your height, weight, or BMI, he or she may ask questions about your health, physical activity, and eating habits. Your doctor also may ask about your family background to find out if you've inherited traits that might make you taller, shorter, or a late bloomer (someone who develops later than other people the same age). The doctor can then put all this information together to decide whether you might have a weight or growth problem.

If your doctor thinks you're overweight, he or she may refer you to a dietitian or doctor specializing in weight management. These experts can offer eating and exercise recommendations based on your individual needs. Following a doctor's or dietitian's plan that's designed especially for you will work way better than following fad diets.

What if you're worried about being too skinny? Most teens who weigh less than other people their age are just fine. You might be going through puberty on a different schedule than some of your peers, and your body may be growing and changing at a different rate. Most underweight teens catch up eventually and there's rarely a need to try to gain weight.

In a few cases, teens can be underweight because of a health problem that needs treatment. See a doctor if you notice any of these things:

- You feel tired or ill a lot.

- You have a cough, stomachache, diarrhea, or other problems that have lasted for more than a week or two.

Some people are underweight because of eating disorders, like anorexia or bulimia, that they need to get help for.

Getting Into Your Genes

Heredity plays a role in body shape and what a person weighs. People from different races, ethnic groups, and nationalities tend to have different body fat distribution (meaning they have fat in different parts of their bodies) or body composition (their amounts of bone and muscle versus fat).

But genes are not destiny. No matter whose genes you inherit, you can have a healthy body and keep your weight at a level that's normal for you by eating right and being active.

Genes aren't the only things that family members may share. Unhealthy eating habits can be passed down, too. The eating and exercise habits of people in the same household may have an even greater effect than genes on a person's risk of becoming overweight.

If your family eats a lot of high-fat foods or snacks or doesn't get much exercise, you may tend to do the same. The good news is these habits can be changed for the better. Even simple changes like walking more or taking the stairs can benefit a person's health.

It can be tough dealing with the physical changes your body goes through during puberty. But at this time, more than any other, it's not a specific number on the scale that's important. It's keeping your body healthy—inside and out.

Chapter 49
Eat The Right Amount Of Calories For You

There's a lot of talk about the different components of food. Whether you're consuming carbohydrates, fats, or proteins all of them contain calories. If your diet focus is on any one of these alone, you're missing the bigger picture.

What Is A Calorie?

A **calorie** is defined as a unit of energy supplied by food. A calorie is a calorie regardless of its source. Whether you're eating carbohydrates, fats, sugars, or proteins, all of them contain calories.

The Caloric Balance Equation

When it comes to maintaining a healthy weight for a lifetime, the bottom line is—**calories count!** Weight management is all about balance—balancing the number of calories you consume with the number of calories your body uses or "burns off."

Caloric balance is like a scale. To remain in balance and maintain your body weight, the calories consumed (from foods) must be balanced by the calories used (in normal body functions, daily activities, and exercise).

About This Chapter: Text in this chapter begins with excerpts from "Finding A Balance," Centers for Disease Control and Prevention (CDC), May 15, 2015; Text under the heading "Estimated Calorie Needs Per Day" is excerpted from "Appendix 2. Estimated Calorie Needs Per Day, By Age, Sex, And Physical Activity Level," Office of Disease Prevention and Health Promotion (ODPHP), U.S. Department of Health and Human Services (HHS), December 15, 2015.

Table 49.1. Caloric Balance Status

If You Are...	Your Caloric Balance Status Is...
Maintaining your weight	**"in balance."** You are eating roughly the same number of calories that your body is using. Your weight will remain **stable**.
Gaining weight	**"in caloric excess."** You are eating more calories than your body is using. You will store these extra calories as fat and you'll **gain** weight.
Losing weight	**"in caloric deficit."** You are eating fewer calories than you are using. Your body is pulling from its fat storage cells for energy, so your weight is **decreasing**.

Am I In Caloric Balance?

If you are maintaining your current body weight, you are in caloric balance. If you need to gain weight or to lose weight, you'll need to tip the balance scale in one direction or another to achieve your goal.

If you need to tip the balance scale in the direction of losing weight, keep in mind that it takes approximately 3,500 calories below your calorie needs to lose a pound of body fat. To lose about 1 to 2 pounds per week, you'll need to reduce your caloric intake by 500–1000 calories per day.

To learn how many calories you are currently eating, begin writing down the foods you eat and the beverages you drink each day. By writing down what you eat and drink, you become more aware of everything you are putting in your mouth. Also, begin writing down the physical activity you do each day and the length of time you do it.

Physical activities (both daily activities and exercise) help tip the balance scale by increasing the calories you expend each day.

Recommended Physical Activity Levels

- 2 hours and 30 minutes (150 minutes) of moderate-intensity aerobic activity (i.e., brisk walking) every week and muscle-strengthening activities on 2 or more days a week that work all major muscle groups (legs, hips, back, abdomen, chest, shoulders, and arms).

- Increasing the intensity or the amount of time that you are physically active can have even greater health benefits and may be needed to control body weight.

- Encourage children and teenagers to be physically active for at least 60 minutes each day, or almost every day.

The bottom line is—each person's body is unique and may have different caloric needs. A healthy lifestyle requires balance, in the foods you eat, in the beverages you consume, in the way you carry out your daily activities, and in the amount of physical activity or exercise you include in your daily routine. While counting calories is not necessary, it may help you in the beginning, to gain an awareness of your eating habits as you strive to achieve energy balance. The ultimate test of balance is whether or not you are gaining, maintaining, or losing weight.

Questions And Answers About Calories

Are Fat-Free And Low-Fat Foods Low In Calories?

Not always. Some fat-free and low-fat foods have extra sugars, which push the calorie amount right back up. The following list of foods and their reduced fat varieties will show you that just because a product is fat-free, it doesn't mean that it is "calorie-free." And, calories do count!

Always read the Nutrition Facts food label to find out the calorie content. Remember, this is the calorie content for one serving of the food item, so be sure and check the serving size. If you eat more than one serving, you'll be eating more calories than is listed on the food label.

If I Eat Late At Night, Will These Calories Automatically Turn Into Body Fat?

The time of day isn't what affects how your body uses calories. It's the overall number of calories you eat and the calories you burn over the course of 24 hours that affects your weight.

I've Heard It Is More Important To Worry About Carbohydrates Than Calories. Is This True?

By focusing only on carbohydrates, you can still eat too many calories. Also, if you drastically reduce the variety of foods in your diet, you could end up sacrificing vital nutrients and not be able to sustain the diet over time.

Does It Matter How Many Calories I Eat As Long As I'm Maintaining An Active Lifestyle

While physical activity is a vital part of weight control, so is controlling the number of calories you eat. If you consume more calories than you use through normal daily activities and physical activity, you will still gain weight.

What Other Factors Contribute To Overweight And Obesity?

Besides diet and behavior, environment, and genetic factors may also have an effect in causing people to be overweight and obese.

Estimated Calorie Needs Per Day

The total number of calories a person needs each day varies depending on a number of factors, including the person's age, sex, height, weight, and level of physical activity. In addition, a need to lose, maintain, or gain weight and other factors affect how many calories should be consumed. Estimated amounts of calories needed to maintain calorie balance for various age and sex groups at three different levels of physical activity are provided in Table 49.2. These estimates are based on the Estimated Energy Requirements (EER) equations, using reference heights (average) and reference weights (healthy) for each age-sex group. For children and adolescents, reference height and weight vary.

Table 49.2. Estimated Calorie Needs Per Day

Male

Age	Sedentary	Moderately active	Active
13	2,000	2,200	2,600
14	2,000	2,400	2,800
15	2,200	2,600	3,000
16	2,400	2,800	3,200
17	2,400	2,800	3,200
18	2,400	2,800	3,200
19-20	2,600	2,800	3,000

Female

Age	Sedentary	Moderately active	Active
13	1,600	2,000	2,200
14	1,800	2,000	2,400
15	1,800	2,000	2,400
16	1,800	2,000	2,400
17	1,800	2,000	2,400
18	1,800	2,000	2,400
19-20	2,000	2,200	2,400

1. Sedentary means a lifestyle that includes only the physical activity of independent living.

2. Moderately Active means a lifestyle that includes physical activity equivalent to walking about 1.5 to 3 miles per day at 3 to 4 miles per hour, in addition to the activities of independent living.

3. Active means a lifestyle that includes physical activity equivalent to walking more than 3 miles per day at 3 to 4 miles per hour, in addition to the activities of independent living.

Chapter 50
Rethink Your Drink

When it comes to weight loss, there's no lack of diets promising fast results. There are low-carb diets, high-carb diets, low-fat diets, grapefruit diets, cabbage soup diets, and blood type diets, to name a few. But no matter what diet you may try, to lose weight, you must take in fewer calories than your body uses. Most people try to reduce their calorie intake by focusing on food, but another way to cut calories may be to think about what you drink.

What Do You Drink? It Makes More Difference Than You Think!

Calories in drinks are not hidden (they're listed right on the Nutrition Facts Label), but many people don't realize just how many calories beverages can contribute to their daily intake. As you can see in the example below, calories from drinks can really add up. But there is good news: you have plenty of options for reducing the number of calories in what you drink.

Table 50.1. Options For Reducing The Number Of Calories

Occasion	Instead Of...	Calories	Try...	Calories
Morning coffee shop run	Medium café latte (16 ounces) made with whole milk	265	Small café latte (12 ounces) made with fat-free milk	125
Lunchtime combo meal	20-oz. bottle of nondiet cola with your lunch	227	Bottle of water or diet soda	0

About This Chapter: This chapter includes text excerpted from "Rethink Your Drink," Centers for Disease Control and Prevention (CDC), September 23, 2015.

Table 50.1. Continued

Occasion	Instead Of...	Calories	Try...	Calories
Afternoon break	Sweetened lemon iced tea from the vending machine (16 ounces)	180	Sparkling water with natural lemon flavor (not sweetened)	0
Dinnertime	A glass of nondiet ginger ale with your meal (12 ounces)	124	Water with a slice of lemon or lime, or seltzer water with a splash of 100 percent fruit juice	0 calories for the water with a fruit slice, or about 30 calories for seltzer water with 2 ounces of 100 percent orange juice.
Total beverage calories:		796		125–155

(USDA National Nutrient Database for Standard Reference)

Substituting no-or low-calorie drinks for sugar-sweetened beverages cuts about 650 calories in the example above.

Of course, not everyone drinks the amount of sugar-sweetened beverages shown above. Check the list below to estimate how many calories you typically take in from beverages.

Table 50.2. Calories For Different Beverages

Type Of Beverage	Calories In 12 Ounces	Calories In 20 Ounces
Fruit punch	192	320
100 percent apple juice	192	300
100 percent orange juice	168	280
Lemonade	168	280
Regular lemon/lime soda	148	247
Regular cola	136	227
Sweetened lemon iced tea (bottled, not homemade)	135	225
Tonic water	124	207
Regular ginger ale	124	207
Sports drink	99	165
Fitness water	18	36
Unsweetened iced tea	2	3

Table 50.2. Continued

Type Of Beverage	Calories In 12 Ounces	Calories In 20 Ounces
Diet soda (with aspartame)	0*	0*
Carbonated water (unsweetened)	0	0
Water	0	0

Some diet soft drinks can contain a small number of calories that are not listed on the nutrition facts label.
(USDA National Nutrient Database for Standard Reference)

Milk contains vitamins and other nutrients that contribute to good health, but it also contains calories. Choosing low-fat or fat-free milk is a good way to reduce your calorie intake and still get the nutrients that milk contains.

Table 50.3. Calories For Different Types Of Milk

Type Of Milk	Calories Per Cup (8 Ounces)
Chocolate milk (whole)	208
Chocolate milk (2 percent reduced-fat)	190
Chocolate milk (1 percent low-fat)	158
Whole Milk (unflavored)	150
2 percent reduced-fat milk (unflavored)	120
1 percent low-fat milk (unflavored)	105
Fat-free milk (unflavored)	90

Some diet soft drinks can contain a small number of calories that are not listed on the nutrition facts label.
(USDA National Nutrient Database for Standard Reference)

Learn To Read Nutrition Facts Labels Carefully

Be aware that the Nutrition Facts label on beverage containers may give the calories for only part of the contents. The example below shows the label on a 20-oz. bottle. As you can see, it lists the number of calories in an 8-oz. serving (100) even though the bottle contains 20 oz. or 2.5 servings. To figure out how many calories are in the whole bottle, you need to multiply the number of calories in one serving by the number of servings in the bottle (100 x 2.5). You can see that the contents of the entire bottle actually contain 250 calories even though what the label calls a "serving" only contains 100. This shows that you need to look closely at the serving size when comparing the calorie content of different beverages.

Sugar By Any Other Name: How To Tell Whether Your Drink Is Sweetened

Sweeteners that add calories to a beverage go by many different names and are not always obvious to anyone looking at the ingredients list. Some common caloric sweeteners are listed below. If these appear in the ingredients list of your favorite beverage, you are drinking a sugar-sweetened beverage.

- High-fructose corn syrup
- Fructose
- Fruit juice concentrates
- Honey
- Sugar
- Syrup
- Corn syrup
- Sucrose
- Dextrose

High-Calorie Culprits In Unexpected Places

Coffee drinks and blended fruit smoothies sound innocent enough, but the calories in some of your favorite coffee-shop or smoothie-stand items may surprise you. Check the website or in-store nutrition information of your favorite coffee or smoothie shop to find out how many calories are in different menu items. And when a smoothie or coffee craving kicks in, here are some tips to help minimize the caloric damage:

At the coffee shop

- Request that your drink be made with fat-free or low-fat milk instead of whole milk
- Order the smallest size available.
- Forgo the extra flavoring—the flavor syrups used in coffee shops, like vanilla or hazelnut, are sugar-sweetened and will add calories to your drink.
- Skip the Whip. The whipped cream on top of coffee drinks adds calories and fat.
- Get back to basics. Order a plain cup of coffee with fat-free milk and artificial sweetener, or drink it black.

At the smoothie stand

- Order a child's size if available.

- Ask to see the nutrition information for each type of smoothie and pick the smoothie with the fewest calories.

- Hold the sugar. Many smoothies contain added sugar in addition to the sugar naturally in fruit, juice, or yogurt. Ask that your smoothie be prepared without added sugar: the fruit is naturally sweet.

Better Beverage Choices Made Easy

Now that you know how much difference a drink can make, here are some ways to make smart beverage choices:

- Choose water, diet, or low-calorie beverages instead of sugar-sweetened beverages.

- For a quick, easy, and inexpensive thirst-quencher, carry a water bottle and refill it throughout the day.

- Don't "stock the fridge" with sugar-sweetened beverages. Instead, keep a jug or bottles of cold water in the fridge.

- Serve water with meals.

- Make water more exciting by adding slices of lemon, lime, cucumber, or watermelon, or drink sparkling water.

- Add a splash of 100 percent juice to plain sparkling water for a refreshing, low-calorie drink.

- When you do opt for a sugar-sweetened beverage, go for the small size. Some companies are now selling 8-oz. cans and bottles of soda, which contain about 100 calories.

- Be a role model for your friends and family by choosing healthy, low-calorie beverages.

Chapter 51

Vegetables And Fruits For A Healthy Weight

How To Use Fruits And Vegetables To Help Manage Your Weight

Fruits and vegetables are part of a well-balanced and healthy eating plan. There are many different ways to lose or maintain a healthy weight. Using more fruits and vegetables along with whole grains and lean meats, nuts, and beans is a safe and healthy one. Helping control your weight is not the only benefit of eating more fruits and vegetables. Diets rich in fruits and vegetables may reduce the risk of some types of cancer and other chronic diseases. Fruits and vegetables also provide essential vitamins and minerals, fiber, and other substances that are important for good health.

To Lose Weight, You Must Eat Fewer Calories Than Your Body Uses

This doesn't necessarily mean that you have to eat less food. You can create lower-calorie versions of some of your favorite dishes by substituting low-calorie fruits and vegetables in place of higher-calorie ingredients. The water and fiber in fruits and vegetables will add volume to your dishes, so you can eat the same amount of food with fewer calories. Most fruits and vegetables are naturally low in fat and calories and are filling.

Here are some simple ways to cut calories and eat fruits and vegetables throughout your day:

About This Chapter: This chapter includes text excerpted from "How To Use Fruits And Vegetables To Help Manage Your Weight," Centers for Disease Control and Prevention (CDC), November 9, 2015.

Breakfast: Start The Day Right

- Substitute some spinach, onions, or mushrooms for one of the eggs or half of the cheese in your morning omelet. The vegetables will add volume and flavor to the dish with fewer calories than the egg or cheese.

- Cut back on the amount of cereal in your bowl to make room for some cut-up bananas, peaches, or strawberries. You can still eat a full bowl, but with fewer calories.

Lighten Up Your Lunch

- Substitute vegetables such as lettuce, tomatoes, cucumbers, or onions for 2 ounces of the cheese and 2 ounces of the meat in your sandwich, wrap, or burrito. The new version will fill you up with fewer calories than the original.

- Add a cup of chopped vegetables, such as broccoli, carrots, beans, or red peppers, in place of 2 ounces of the meat or 1 cup of noodles in your favorite broth-based soup. The vegetables will help fill you up, so you won't miss those extra calories.

Dinner

- Add in 1 cup of chopped vegetables such as broccoli, tomatoes, squash, onions, or peppers, while removing 1 cup of the rice or pasta in your favorite dish. The dish with the vegetables will be just as satisfying but have fewer calories than the same amount of the original version.

- Take a good look at your dinner plate. Vegetables, fruit, and whole grains should take up the largest portion of your plate. If they do not, replace some of the meat, cheese, white pasta, or rice with legumes, steamed broccoli, asparagus, greens, or another favorite vegetable. This will reduce the total calories in your meal without reducing the amount of food you eat. BUT remember to use a normal-or small-size plate—not a platter. The total number of calories that you eat counts, even if a good proportion of them come from fruits and vegetables.

Smart Snacks

- Most healthy eating plans allow for one or two small snacks a day. Choosing most fruits and vegetables will allow you to eat a snack with only 100 calories.

- Instead of a high-calorie snack from a vending machine, bring some cut-up vegetables or fruit from home. One snack-sized bag of corn chips (1 ounce) has the same number of calories as a small apple, 1 cup of whole strawberries, AND 1 cup of carrots with 1/4 cup of low-calorie dip. Substitute one or two of these options for the chips, and you will have a satisfying snack with fewer calories.

About 100 Calories Or Less
- a medium-size apple (72 calories)
- a medium-size banana (105 calories)
- 1 cup steamed green beans (44 calories)
- 1 cup blueberries (83 calories)
- 1 cup grapes (100 calories)
- 1 cup carrots (45 calories), broccoli (30 calories), or bell peppers (30 calories) with 2 tbsp. hummus (46 calories)

Remember: Substitution Is The Key

It's true that fruits and vegetables are lower in calories than many other foods, but they do contain some calories. If you start eating fruits and vegetables in addition to what you usually eat, you are adding calories and may gain weight. The key is the substitution. Eat fruits and vegetables instead of some other higher-calorie food.

More Tips For Making Fruits And Vegetables Part Of Your Weight Management Plan

Eat fruits and vegetables the way nature provided—or with fat-free or low-fat cooking techniques.

Try steaming your vegetables, using low-calorie or low-fat dressings, and using herbs and spices to add flavor. Some cooking techniques, such as breading and frying, or using high-fat dressings or sauces will greatly increase the calories and fat in the dish. And eat your fruit raw to enjoy its natural sweetness.

Canned or frozen fruits and vegetables are also good options.

Frozen or canned fruits and vegetables can be just as nutritious as the fresh varieties. However, be careful to choose those without added sugar, syrup, cream sauces, or other ingredients that will add calories.

Choose whole fruit over fruit drinks and juices. Fruit juices have lost fiber from the fruit.

It is better to eat the whole fruit because it contains the added fiber that helps you feel full. One 6-ounce serving of orange juice has 85 calories, compared to just 65 calories in a medium orange.

Whole fruit gives you a bigger size snack than the same fruit dried—for the same number of calories.

A small box of raisins (1/4 cup) is about 100 calories. For the same number of calories, you can eat 1 cup of grapes.

Chapter 52

How To Choose A Safe Weight-Loss Program

Do you need to lose weight?

Have you been thinking about trying a weight-loss program?

Diets and programs that promise to help you lose weight are advertised everywhere—through magazines and newspapers, radio, TV, and websites. Are these programs safe? Will they work for you?

This chapter provides tips on how to identify a weight-loss program that may help you lose weight safely and keep the weight off over time. It also suggests ways to talk to your healthcare provider about your weight. He or she may be able to help you control your weight by making changes to your eating and physical activity habits. If these changes are not enough, you may want to consider a weight-loss program or other types of treatment.

Where Do I Start?

Talking to your healthcare provider about your weight is an important first step. Doctors do not always address issues such as healthy eating, physical activity, and weight control during general office visits. It is important for you to bring up these issues to get the help you need. Even if you feel uneasy talking about your weight with your doctor, remember that he or she is there to help you improve your health.

Prepare for the visit:

- Write down your questions in advance.

About This Chapter: This chapter includes text excerpted from "Choosing A Safe And Successful Weight-Loss Program," National Institute of Diabetes and Digestive and Kidney Diseases (NIDDK), December 2012. Reviewed March 2017.

- Bring pen and paper to take notes.

- Invite a family member or friend along for support if this will make you feel better.

Talk to your doctor about safe and effective ways to control your weight.

He or she can review any medical problems that you have and any drugs that you take to help you set goals for controlling your weight. Make sure you understand what your doctor is saying. Ask questions if you do not understand something.

You may want to ask your doctor to recommend a weight-loss program or specialist. If you do start a weight-loss program, discuss your choice of program with your doctor, especially if you have any health problems.

Questions To Ask Your Healthcare Provider

About your weight

- What is a healthy weight for me?
- Do I need to lose weight?
- How much weight should I lose?
- Could my extra weight be caused by a health problem or by a medicine I am taking?

About ways to lose weight

- What kind of eating habits may help me control my weight?
- How much physical activity do I need?
- How can I exercise safely?
- Could a weight-loss program help me?
- Should I take weight-loss drugs?
- Is weight-loss surgery right for me?

What Should I Look For In A Weight-Loss Program?

Successful, long-term weight control must focus on your overall health, not just on what you eat. Changing your lifestyle is not easy, but adopting healthy habits may help you manage your weight in the long run.

Effective weight-loss programs include ways to keep the weight off for good. These programs promote healthy behaviors that help you lose weight and that you can stick with every day.

Safe and effective weight-loss programs should include:

- a plan to keep the weight off over the long run

- guidance on how to develop healthier eating and physical activity habits

- ongoing feedback, monitoring, and support

- slow and steady weight-loss goals—usually ½ to 2 pounds per week (though weight loss may be faster at the start of a program)

Some weight-loss programs may use very low-calorie diets (up to 800 calories per day) to promote rapid weight loss among people who have a lot of excess weight. This type of diet requires close medical supervision through frequent office visits and medical tests.

What If The Program Is Offered Online?

Many weight-loss programs are now being offered online—either fully or partly. Not much is known about how well these programs work. However, experts suggest that online weight-loss programs should provide the following:

- structured, weekly lessons offered online or by podcasts support tailored to your personal goals

- support tailored to your personal goals

- self-monitoring of eating and physical activity using handheld devices, such as cell phones or online journals

- regular feedback from a counselor on goals, progress, and results, given by email, phone, or text messages

- social support from a group through bulletin boards, chat rooms, and/or online meetings

Whether the program is online or in person, you should get as much background as you can before deciding to join.

What Questions Should I Ask About The Program?

Professionals working for weight-loss programs should be able to answer questions about the program's features, safety, costs, and results. The following are sample questions you may want to ask.

What Does The Weight-Loss Program Include?

- Does the program offer group classes or one-on-one counseling that will help me develop healthier habits?

- Do I have to follow a specific meal plan or keep food records?

- Do I have to buy special meals or supplements?

- If the program requires special foods, can I make changes based on my likes, dislikes, and food allergies (if any)?

- Will the program help me be more physically active, follow a specific physical activity plan, or provide exercise guidelines?

- Will the program work with my lifestyle and cultural needs? Does the program provide ways to deal with such issues as social or holiday eating, changes to work schedules, lack of motivation, and injury or illness?

- Does the program include a plan to help me keep the weight off once I've lost weight?

What Are The Staff Credentials?

- Who supervises the program?

- What type of weight-control certifications, education, experience, and training do the staff have?

Does The Product Or Program Carry Any Risks?

- Could the program hurt me?

- Could the suggested drugs or supplements harm my health?

- Do the people involved in the program get to talk with a doctor?

- Does a doctor or other certified health professional run the program?

- Will the program's doctor or staff work with my healthcare provider if needed (for example, to address how the program may affect an existing medical issue)?

- Is there ongoing input and follow-up from a healthcare provider to ensure my safety while I take part in the program?

How Much Does The Program Cost?

- What is the total cost of the program?

- Are there other costs, such as membership fees, fees for weekly visits, and payments for food, meal replacements, supplements, or other products?

- Are there other fees for medical tests?

- Are there fees for a follow-up program after I lose weight?

What Results Do People In The Program Typically Have?

- How much weight does the average person lose?

- How long does the average person keep the weight off?

- Do you have written information on these results?

If It Seems Too Good To Be True...It Probably Is!

In choosing a weight-loss program, watch out for these false claims:

- Lose weight without diet or exercise!
- Lose weight while eating all of your favorite foods!
- Lose 30 pounds in 30 days!
- Lose weight in specific problem areas of your body!

Other warning signs include:

- very small print
- asterisks and footnotes
- before-and-after photos that seem too good to be true

For more background on false claims used by some weight-loss programs and products, see the items from the Federal Trade Commission listed in the For More Information section.

Chapter 53
Healthy Eating For Vegetarians

Vegetarian diets can meet all the recommendations for nutrients. The key is to consume a variety of foods and the right amount of foods to meet your calorie needs. Follow the food group recommendations for your age, sex, and activity level to get the right amount of food and the variety of foods needed for nutrient adequacy. Nutrients that vegetarians may need to focus on include protein, iron, calcium, zinc, and vitamin B12.

Nutrients To Focus On For Vegetarians

* **Protein** has many important functions in the body and is essential for growth and mainte-nance. Protein needs can easily be met by eating a variety of plant-based foods. Combining different protein sources in the same meal is not necessary. Sources of protein for vegetari-ans and vegans include beans, nuts, nut butters, peas, and soy products (tofu, tempeh, veggie burgers). Milk products and eggs are also good protein sources for lacto-ovo vegetarians.

* **Iron** functions primarily as a carrier of oxygen in the blood. Iron sources for vegetarians and vegans include iron-fortified breakfast cereals, spinach, kidney beans, black-eyed peas, lentils, turnip greens, molasses, whole wheat breads, peas, and some dried fruits (dried apricots, prunes, raisins).

* **Calcium** is used for building bones and teeth and in maintaining bone strength. Sources of calcium for vegetarians and vegans include calcium-fortified soymilk, calcium-fortified

About This Chapter: Text in this chapter begins with excerpts from "Tips For Vegetarians," ChooseMyPlate. gov, U.S. Department of Agriculture (USDA), October 12, 2016; Text under the heading "Healthy Vegetarian Eating Pattern" is excerpted from "Appendix 5. USDA Food Patterns: Healthy Vegetarian Eating Pattern," Office of Disease Prevention and Health Promotion (ODPHP), U.S. Department of Health and Human Services (HHS), December 15, 2015.

breakfast cereals and orange juice, tofu made with calcium sulfate, and some dark-green leafy vegetables (collard greens, turnip greens, bok choy, mustard greens). The amount of calcium that can be absorbed from these foods varies. Consuming enough plant foods to meet calcium needs may be unrealistic for many. Milk products are excellent calcium sources for lacto vegetarians. Calcium supplements are another potential source.

- **Zinc** is necessary for many biochemical reactions and also helps the immune system function properly. Sources of zinc for vegetarians and vegans include many types of beans (white beans, kidney beans, and chickpeas), zinc-fortified breakfast cereals, wheat germ, and pumpkin seeds. Milk products are a zinc source for lacto vegetarians.

- **Vitamin B12** is found in animal products and some fortified foods. Sources of vitamin B12 for vegetarians include milk products, eggs, and foods that have been fortified with vitamin B12. These include breakfast cereals, soymilk, veggie burgers, and nutritional yeast.

Tips For Vegetarians

- Build meals around protein sources that are naturally low in fat, such as beans, lentils, and rice. Don't overload meals with high-fat cheeses to replace the meat.

- Calcium-fortified soy milk provides calcium in amounts similar to milk. It is usually low in fat and does not contain cholesterol.

- Many foods that typically contain meat or poultry can be made vegetarian. This can increase vegetable intake and cut saturated fat and cholesterol intake. Consider:

  - pasta primavera or pasta with marinara or pesto sauce

  - veggie pizza

  - vegetable lasagna

  - tofu-vegetable stir fry

  - vegetable lo mein

  - vegetable kabobs

  - bean burritos or tacos

- A variety of vegetarian products look (and may taste) like their non-vegetarian counterparts, but are usually lower in saturated fat and contain no cholesterol.

- For breakfast, try soy-based sausage patties or links.

- Rather than hamburgers, try veggie burgers. A variety of kinds are available, made with soy beans, vegetables, and/or rice.

- Add vegetarian meat substitutes to soups and stews to boost protein without adding saturated fat or cholesterol. These include tempeh (cultured soybeans with a chewy texture), tofu, or wheat gluten (seitan).

- For barbecues, try veggie burgers, soy hot dogs, marinated tofu or tempeh, and veggie kabobs.

- Make bean burgers, lentil burgers, or pita halves with falafel (spicy ground chickpea patties).

- Some restaurants offer soy options (texturized vegetable protein) as a substitute for meat, and soy cheese as a substitute for regular cheese.

- Most restaurants can accommodate vegetarian modifications to menu items by substituting meatless sauces, omitting meat from stir-fries, and adding vegetables or pasta in place of meat. These substitutions are more likely to be available at restaurants that make food to order.

- Many Asian and Indian restaurants offer a varied selection of vegetarian dishes.

Healthy Vegetarian Eating Pattern

The Healthy Vegetarian Pattern is adapted from the Healthy U.S.-Style Pattern, modifying amounts recommended from some food groups to more closely reflect eating patterns reported by self-identified vegetarians in the National Health and Nutrition Examination Survey (NHANES). This analysis allowed development of a Pattern that is based on evidence of the foods and amounts consumed by vegetarians, in addition to meeting the same nutrient and Dietary Guidelines standards as the Healthy U.S.-Style Pattern. Based on a comparison of the food choices of these vegetarians to nonvegetarians in NHANES, amounts of soy products (particularly tofu and other processed soy products), legumes, nuts and seeds, and whole grains were increased, and meat, poultry, and seafood were eliminated. Dairy and eggs were included because they were consumed by the majority of these vegetarians. This Pattern can be vegan if all dairy choices are comprised of fortified soy beverages (soymilk) or other plant-based dairy substitutes. Note that vegetarian adaptations of the USDA Food Patterns were included in the 2010 Dietary Guidelines. However, those adaptations did not modify the underlying structure of the Patterns, but substituted the same amounts of plant foods for animal foods in each food group. In contrast, the current Healthy Vegetarian Pattern includes changes in food group composition and amounts, based on assessing the food choices of vegetarians. The Pattern is similar in meeting nutrient standards to the Healthy U.S.-Style Pattern, but somewhat higher in calcium and fiber and lower in vitamin D due to differences in the foods included.

To follow this Pattern, identify the appropriate calorie level, choose a variety of foods in each group and subgroup over time in recommended amounts, and limit choices that are not in nutrient-dense forms so that the overall calorie limit is not exceeded.

Table 53.1. Healthy Vegetarian Eating Pattern: Recommended Amounts Of Food From Each Food Group

Calorie Level of Pattern	1,000	1,200	1,400	1,600	1,800	2,000
Food Group	**Daily Amount of Food From Each Group (vegetable and protein foods subgroup amounts are per week)**					
Vegetables	1 c-eq	1½ c-eq	1½ c-eq	2 c-eq	2½ c-eq	2½ c-eq
Dark-green vegetables (c-eq/wk)	½	1	1	1½	1½	1½
Red and orange vegetables (c-eq/wk)	2½	3	3	4	5½	5½
Legumes (beans and peas) (c-eq/wk)d	½	½	½	1	1½	1½
Starchy vegetables (c-eq/wk)	2	3½	3½	4	5	5
Other vegetables (c-eq/wk)	1½	2½	2½	3½	4	4
Fruits	1 c-eq	1 c-eq	1½ c-eq	1½ c-eq	1½ c-eq	2 c-eq
Grains	3 oz-eq	4 oz-eq	5 oz-eq	5½ oz-eq	6½ oz-eq	6½ oz-eq
Whole grains (oz-eq/day)	1½	2	2½	3	3½	3½
Refined grains (oz-eq/day)	1½	2	2½	2½	3	3
Dairy	2 c-eq	2.5 c-eq	2.5 c-eq	3 c-eq	3 c-eq	3 c-eq
Protein Foods	1 oz-eq	1½ oz-eq	2 oz-eq	2½ oz-eq	3 oz-eq	3½ oz-eq
Eggs (oz-eq/wk)	2	3	3	3	3	3
Legumes (beans and peas) (oz-eq/wk)d	1	2	4	4	6	6
Soy products (oz-eq/wk)	2	3	4	6	6	8
Nuts and seeds (oz-eq/wk)	2	2	3	5	6	7
Oils	15 g	17 g	17 g	22 g	24 g	27 g
Limit on Calories for Other Uses, calories (% of calories)	190 (19%)	170 (14%)	190 (14%)	180 (11%)	190 (11%)	290 (15%)

Chapter 54
Healthy Eating For Athletes

Eat Extra For Excellence

There's a lot more to eating for sports than chowing down on carbs or chugging sports drinks. The good news is that eating to reach your peak performance level likely doesn't require a special diet or supplements. It's all about working the right foods into your fitness plan in the right amounts.

Teen athletes have unique nutritional needs. Because athletes work out more than their less-active peers, they generally need extra calories to fuel both their sports performance and their growth. Depending on how active they are, teen athletes may need anywhere from 2,000 to 5,000 total calories per day to meet their energy needs.

So what happens if teen athletes don't eat enough? Their bodies are less likely to achieve peak performance and may even break down rather than build up muscles. Athletes who don't take in enough calories every day won't be as fast and as strong as they could be and may not be able to maintain their weight. And extreme calorie restriction can lead to growth problems and other serious health risks for both girls and guys, including increased risk for fractures and other injuries.

Athletes And Dieting

Since teen athletes need extra fuel, it's usually a bad idea to diet. Athletes in sports where weight is emphasized—such as wrestling, swimming, dance, or gymnastics—might feel

About This Chapter: Text in this chapter is © 1995-2017. The Nemours Foundation/KidsHealth®. Reprinted with permission.

pressure to lose weight, but they need to balance that choice with the possible negative side effects mentioned above.

If a coach, gym teacher, or teammate says that you need to go on a diet, talk to your doctor first or visit a dietitian who specializes in teen athletes. If a health professional you trust agrees that it's safe to diet, then he or she can work with you to develop a plan that allows you get the proper amount of nutrients, and perform your best while also losing weight.

Eat A Variety Of Foods

You may have heard about "carb loading" before a game. But when it comes to powering your game for the long haul, it's a bad idea to focus on only one type of food.

Carbohydrates are an important source of fuel, but they're only one of many foods an athlete needs. It also takes vitamins, minerals, protein, and fats to stay in peak playing shape.

Muscular Minerals And Vital Vitamins

Calcium helps build the strong bones that athletes depend on, and iron carries oxygen to muscles. Most teens don't get enough of these minerals, and that's especially true of teen athletes because their needs may be even higher than those of other teens.

To get the iron you need, eat lean (not much fat) meat, fish, and poultry; green, leafy vegetables; and iron-fortified cereals. Calcium—a must for protecting against stress fractures—is found in dairy foods, such as low-fat milk, yogurt, and cheese.

In addition to calcium and iron, you need a whole bunch of other vitamins and minerals that do everything from help you access energy to keep you from getting sick. Eating a balanced diet, including lots of different fruits and veggies, should provide the vitamins and minerals needed for good health and sports performance.

Protein Power

Athletes may need more protein than less-active teens, but most teen athletes get plenty of protein through regular eating. It's a myth that athletes need a huge daily intake of protein to build large, strong muscles. Muscle growth comes from regular training and hard work. And taking in too much protein can actually harm the body, causing dehydration, calcium loss, and even kidney problems.

Good sources of protein are fish, lean meats and poultry, eggs, dairy, nuts, soy, and peanut butter.

Carb Charge

Carbohydrates provide athletes with an excellent source of fuel. Cutting back on carbs or following low-carb diets isn't a good idea for athletes because restricting carbohydrates can cause a person to feel tired and worn out, which ultimately affects performance.

Good sources of carbohydrates include fruits, vegetables, and grains. Choose whole grains (such as brown rice, oatmeal, whole-wheat bread) more often than their more processed counterparts like white rice and white bread. That's because whole grains provide both the energy athletes need to perform and the fiber and other nutrients they need to be healthy.

Sugary carbs such as candy bars or sodas are less healthy for athletes because they don't contain any of the other nutrients you need. In addition, eating candy bars or other sugary snacks just before practice or competition can give athletes a quick burst of energy and then leave them to "crash" or run out of energy before they've finished working out.

Fat Fuel

Everyone needs a certain amount of fat each day, and this is particularly true for athletes. That's because active muscles quickly burn through carbs and need fats for long-lasting energy. Like carbs, not all fats are created equal. Experts advise athletes to concentrate on eating healthier fats, such as the unsaturated fat found in most vegetable oils, some fish, and nuts and seeds. Try to not to eat too much trans fat—like partially hydrogenated oils—and saturated fat, that is found in high fat meat and high fat dairy products, like butter.

Choosing when to eat fats is also important for athletes. Fatty foods can slow digestion, so it's a good idea to avoid eating these foods for a few hours before and after exercising.

Shun Supplements

Protein and energy bars don't do a whole lot of good, but they won't really do you much harm either. Energy drinks have lots of caffeine, though, so no one should drink them before exercising.

Other types of supplements can really do some damage.

Anabolic steroids can seriously mess with a person's hormones, causing side effects like testicular shrinkage and baldness in guys and facial hair growth in girls. Steroids can cause mental health problems, including depression and serious mood swings.

Some supplements contain hormones that are related to testosterone (such as dehydroepi-androsterone, or DHEA for short). These supplements can have similar side effects to anabolic steroids. Other sports supplements (like creatine, for example) have not been tested in people younger than 18. So the risks of taking them are not yet known.

Salt tablets are another supplement to watch out for. People take them to avoid dehydration, but salt tablets can actually lead to dehydration. In large amounts, salt can cause nausea, vomiting, cramps, and diarrhea and may damage the lining of the stomach. In general, you are better off drinking fluids in order to maintain hydration. Any salt you lose in sweat can usually be made up with sports drinks or food eaten after exercise.

Ditch Dehydration

Speaking of dehydration, water is just as important to unlocking your game power as food. When you sweat during exercise, it's easy to become overheated, headachy, and worn out—especially in hot or humid weather. Even mild dehydration can affect an athlete's physical and mental performance.

There's no one-size-fits-all formula for how much water to drink. How much fluid each person needs depends on the individual's age, size, level of physical activity, and environmental temperature.

Experts recommend that athletes drink before and after exercise as well as every 15 to 20 minutes during exercise. Don't wait until you feel thirsty, because thirst is a sign that your body has needed liquids for a while. But don't force yourself to drink more fluids than you may need either. It's hard to run when there's a lot of water sloshing around in your stomach!

If you like the taste of sports drinks better than regular water, then it's OK to drink them. But it's important to know that a sports drink is really no better for you than water unless you are exercising for more than 60 to 90 minutes or in really hot weather. The additional carbohydrates and electrolytes may improve performance in these conditions, but otherwise your body will do just as well with water.

Avoid drinking carbonated drinks or juice because they could give you a stomachache while you're competing.

Never drink energy drinks before exercising. Energy drinks contain a large amount of caffeine and other ingredients that have caffeine-like effects.

Caffeine

Caffeine is a diuretic. That means it causes a person to urinate (pee) more. It's not clear whether this causes dehydration or not, but to be safe, it's wise to stay away from too much caffeine. That's especially true if you'll be exercising in hot weather.

When it comes to caffeine and exercise, it's good to weigh any benefits against potential problems. Although some studies find that caffeine may help adults perform better in endurance sports, other studies show too much caffeine may hurt.

Caffeine increases heart rate and blood pressure. Too much caffeine can leave an athlete feeling anxious or jittery. Caffeine can also cause trouble sleeping. All of these can drag down a person's sports performance. Plus, taking certain medications—including supplements—can make caffeine's side effects seem even worse.

Never drink energy drinks before exercising. These products contain a large amount of caffeine and other ingredients that have caffeine-like effects.

Game-Day Eats

Your performance on game day will depend on the foods you've eaten over the past several days and weeks. But you can boost your performance even more by paying attention to the food you eat on game day. Strive for a game-day diet rich in carbohydrates, moderate in protein, and low in fat.

Here are some guidelines on what to eat and when:

- **Eat a meal 2 to 4 hours before the game or event:** Choose a protein and carbohydrate meal (like a turkey or chicken sandwich, cereal and milk, chicken noodle soup and yogurt, or pasta with tomato sauce).

- **Eat a snack less than 2 hours before the game:** If you haven't had time to have a pregame meal, be sure to have a light snack such as low-fiber fruits or vegetables (like plums, melons, cherries, carrots), crackers, a bagel, or low-fat yogurt.

Consider not eating anything for the hour before you compete or have practice because digestion requires energy—energy that you want to use to win. Also, eating too soon before any kind of activity can leave food in the stomach, making you feel full, bloated, crampy, and sick.

Everyone is different, so get to know what works best for you. You may want to experiment with meal timing and how much to eat on practice days so that you're better prepared for game day.

Want to get an eating plan personalized for you? The U.S. government's website ChooseMyPlate.gov, tells a person how much to eat from different food groups based on age, gender, and activity level.

Chapter 55

Physical Fitness For Teens

What Is Physical Activity?

Physical activity simply means movement of the body that uses energy. Walking, gardening, briskly pushing a baby stroller, climbing the stairs, playing soccer, or dancing the night away are all good examples of being active. For health benefits, physical activity should be moderate or vigorous intensity

Why Do We Need Physical Activity?

Regular physical activity is important for good health, and it's especially important if you're trying to lose weight or to maintain a healthy weight.

- When losing weight, more physical activity increases the number of calories your body uses for energy or "burns off." The burning of calories through physical activity, combined with reducing the number of calories you eat, creates a "calorie deficit" that results in weight loss.

- Most weight loss occurs because of decreased caloric intake. However, evidence shows the only way to maintain weight loss is to be engaged in regular physical activity.

- Most importantly, physical activity reduces risks of cardiovascular disease and diabetes beyond that produced by weight reduction alone.

About This Chapter: Text under the heading "What Is Physical Activity?" is excerpted from "Physical Activity," ChooseMyPlate.gov, U.S. Department of Agriculture (USDA), June 10, 2015; Text under the heading "Why Do We Need Physical Activity?" excerpted from "Physical Activity for a Healthy Weight," Centers for Disease Control and Prevention (CDC), May 15, 2015; Text under the heading "Active Children And Adolescents" is excerpted from "Chapter 3: Active Children And Adolescents," Office of Disease Prevention and Health Promotion (ODPHP), U.S. Department of Health and Human Services (HHS), February 16, 2017.

Physical activity also helps to:

- Maintain weight.

- Reduce high blood pressure.

- Reduce risk for type 2 diabetes, heart attack, stroke, and several forms of cancer.

- Reduce arthritis pain and associated disability.

- Reduce risk for osteoporosis and falls.

- Reduce symptoms of depression and anxiety.

Active Children And Adolescents

Regular physical activity in children and adolescents promotes health and fitness. Compared to those who are inactive, physically active youth have higher levels of cardiorespiratory fitness and stronger muscles. They also typically have lower body fatness. Their bones are stronger, and they may have reduced symptoms of anxiety and depression.

Youth who are regularly active also have a better chance of a healthy adulthood. Children and adolescents don't usually develop chronic diseases, such as heart disease, hypertension, type 2 diabetes, or osteoporosis. However, risk factors for these diseases can begin to develop early in life. Regular physical activity makes it less likely that these risk factors will develop and more likely that children will remain healthy as adults.

Youth can achieve substantial health benefits by doing moderate- and vigorous-intensity physical activity for periods of time that add up to 60 minutes (1 hour) or more each day. This activity should include aerobic activity as well as age-appropriate muscle- and bone–strengthening activities. Although current science is not complete, it appears that, as with adults, the total amount of physical activity is more important for achieving health benefits than is any one component (frequency, intensity, or duration) or specific mix of activities (aerobic, muscle-strengthening, bone strengthening). Even so, bone-strengthening activities remain especially important for children and young adolescents because the greatest gains in bone mass occur during the years just before and during puberty. In addition, the majority of peak bone mass is obtained by the end of adolescence.

This chapter provides physical activity guidance for children and adolescents aged 6 to 17, and focuses on physical activity beyond baseline activity.

Parents and other adults who work with or care for youth should be familiar with the Guidelines in this chapter. These adults should be aware that, as children become adolescents, they typically reduce their physical activity. Adults play an important role in providing age-appropriate opportunities for physical activity. In doing so, they help lay an important foundation for lifelong, health-promoting physical activity. Adults need to encourage active play in children and encourage sustained and structured activity as children grow older.

Key Guidelines For Children And Adolescents

- Children and adolescents should do 60 minutes (1 hour) or more of physical activity daily.
  - **Aerobic.** Most of the 60 or more minutes a day should be either moderate- or vigorous-intensity aerobic physical activity, and should include vigorous-intensity physical activity at least 3 days a week.
  - **Muscle-strengthening.** As part of their 60 or more minutes of daily physical activity, children and adolescents should include muscle-strengthening physical activity on at least 3 days of the week.
  - **Bone-strengthening.** As part of their 60 or more minutes of daily physical activity, children and adolescents should include bone-strengthening physical activity on at least 3 days of the week.
- It is important to encourage young people to participate in physical activities that are appropriate for their age, that are enjoyable, and that offer variety.

Explaining The Guidelines

Types Of Activity

The Guidelines for children and adolescents focus on three types of activity: aerobic, muscle-strengthening, and bone-strengthening. Each type has important health benefits.

- **Aerobic activities** are those in which young people rhythmically move their large muscles. Running, hopping, skipping, jumping rope, swimming, dancing, and bicycling are all examples of aerobic activities. Aerobic activities increase cardiorespiratory fitness. Children often do activities in short bursts, which may not technically be aerobic activities. However, this document will also use the term aerobic to refer to these brief activities.

- **Muscle-strengthening activities** make muscles do more work than usual during activities of daily life. This is called "overload," and it strengthens the muscles.

Muscle-strengthening activities can be unstructured and part of play, such as playing on playground equipment, climbing trees, and playing tug-of-war. Or these activities can be structured, such as lifting weights or working with resistance bands.

- **Bone-strengthening activities** produce a force on the bones that promotes bone growth and strength. This force is commonly produced by impact with the ground. Running, jumping rope, basketball, tennis, and hopscotch are all examples of bone strengthening activities. As these examples illustrate, bone-strengthening activities can also be aerobic and muscle-strengthening.

How Age Influences Physical Activity In Children And Adolescents

Children and adolescents should meet the Guidelines by doing activity that is appropriate for their age. Their natural patterns of movement differ from those of adults. For example, children are naturally active in an intermittent way, particularly when they do unstructured active play. During recess and in their free play and games, children use basic aerobic and bone-strengthening activities, such as running, hopping, skipping, and jumping, to develop movement patterns and skills. They alternate brief periods of moderate- and vigorous-intensity physical activity with brief periods of rest. Any episode of moderate-or vigorous–intensity physical activity, however brief, counts toward the Guidelines.

Children also commonly increase muscle strength through unstructured activities that involve lifting or moving their body weight or working against resistance. Children don't usually do or need formal muscle-strengthening programs, such as lifting weights.

> Regular physical activity in children and adolescents promotes a healthy body weight and body composition.

As children grow into adolescents, their patterns of physical activity change. They are able to play organized games and sports and are able to sustain longer periods of activity. But they still commonly do an intermittent activity, and no period of moderate- or vigorous-intensity activity is too short to count toward the Guidelines.

Adolescents may meet the Guidelines by doing free play, structured programs, or both. Structured exercise programs can include aerobic activities, such as playing a sport, and muscle-strengthening activities, such as lifting weights, working with resistance bands, or using body weight for resistance (such as push-ups, pull-ups, and sit-ups). Muscle-strengthening activities count if they involve a moderate to high level of effort and work the major muscle groups of the body: legs, hips, back, abdomen, chest, shoulders, and arms.

Levels Of Intensity For Aerobic Activity

Children and adolescents can meet the Guidelines by doing a combination of moderate and vigorous-intensity aerobic physical activities or by doing only vigorous-intensity aerobic physical activities.

Youth should not do only moderate-intensity activity. It's important to include vigorous-intensity activities because they cause more improvement in cardiorespiratory fitness.

The intensity of aerobic physical activity can be defined on either an absolute or a relative scale. Either scale can be used to monitor the intensity of aerobic physical activity:

- **Absolute intensity** is based on the rate of energy expenditure during the activity, without taking into account a person's cardiorespiratory fitness.

- **Relative intensity** uses a person's level of cardiorespiratory fitness to assess the level of effort.

Relative intensity describes a person's level of effort relative to his or her fitness. As a rule of thumb, on a scale of 0 to 10, where sitting is 0 and the highest level of effort possible is 10, moderate-intensity activity is a 5 or 6. Young people doing moderate-intensity activity will notice that their hearts are beating faster than normal and they are breathing harder than normal. Vigorous-intensity activity is at a level of 7 or 8. Youth doing vigorous-intensity activity will feel their heart beating much faster than normal and they will breathe much harder than normal.

When adults supervise children, they generally can't ascertain a child's heart or breathing rate. But they can observe whether a child is doing an activity which, based on absolute energy expenditure, is considered to be either moderate or vigorous. For example, a child walking briskly to school is a moderate-intensity activity. A child running on the playground is doing a vigorous-intensity activity. The table below includes examples of activities classified by absolute intensity. It shows that the same activity can be moderate or vigorous intensity, depending on factors such as speed (for example bicycling slowly or fast).

Table 55.1. Examples Of Moderate-And Vigorous-Intensity Aerobic Physical Activities And Muscle-And Bone-strengthening Activities For Children And Adolescents

Type Of Physical Activity	Age Group Children	Age Group Adults
Moderate–intensity aerobic	• Active recreation, such as hiking, skateboarding, rollerblading • Bicycle riding • Brisk walking	• Active recreation, such as canoeing, hiking, skateboarding, rollerblading • Brisk walking • Bicycle riding (stationary or road bike) • Housework and yard work, such as sweeping or pushing a lawn mower • Games that require catching and throwing, such as baseball and softball
Vigorous–intensity aerobic	• Active games involving running and chasing, such as tag • Bicycle riding • Jumping rope • Martial arts, such as karate • Running • Sports such as soccer, ice or field hockey, basketball, swimming, tennis • Cross-country skiing	• Active games involving running and chasing, such as flag football • Bicycle riding • Jumping rope • Martial arts, such as karate • Running • Sports such as soccer, ice or field hockey, basketball, swimming, tennis • Vigorous dancing • Cross-country skiing
Muscle-strengthening	• Games such as tug-of-war • Modified push-ups (with knees on the floor) • Resistance exercises using body weight or resistance bands • Rope or tree climbing • Sit-ups (curl-ups or crunches) • Swinging on playground equipment/bars	• Games such as tug-of-war • Push-ups and pull-ups • Resistance exercises with exercise bands, weight machines, hand-held weights • Climbing wall • Sit-ups (curl-ups or crunches)

Table 55.1. Continued

Type Of Physical Activity	Age Group Children	Age Group Adults
Bone-strengthening	• Games such as hopscotch • Hopping, skipping, jumping • Jumping rope • Running • Sports such as gymnastics, basketball, volleyball, tennis	• Hopping, skipping, jumping • Jumping rope • Running • Sports such as gymnastics, basketball, volleyball, tennis

Note: Some activities, such as bicycling, can be moderate or vigorous intensity, depending upon level of effort

Physical Activity And Healthy Weight

Regular physical activity in children and adolescents promotes a healthy body weight and body composition.

Exercise training in overweight or obese youth can improve body composition by reducing overall levels of fatness as well as abdominal fatness. Research studies report that fatness can be reduced by a regular physical activity of moderate to vigorous intensity 3 to 5 times a week, for 30 to 60 minutes.

Meeting The Guidelines

American youth vary in their physical activity participation. Some don't participate at all, others participate in enough activity to meet the Guidelines, and some exceed the Guidelines.

> Children and adolescents can meet the Physical Activity Guidelines and become regularly physically active in many ways.

One practical strategy to promote activity in youth is to replace inactivity with activity whenever possible. For example, where appropriate and safe, young people should walk or bicycle to school instead of riding in a car. Rather than just watching sporting events on television, young people should participate in age-appropriate sports or games.

- **Children and adolescents who do not meet the Guidelines** should slowly increase their activity in small steps and in ways that they enjoy. A gradual increase in the number of days and the time spent being active will help reduce the risk of injury.

- **Children and adolescents who meet the Guidelines** should continue being active on a daily basis and, if appropriate, become even more active. Evidence suggests that even more than 60 minutes of activity every day may provide additional health benefits.

- **Children and adolescents who exceed the Guidelines** should maintain their activity level and vary the kinds of activities they do to reduce the risk of overtraining or injury.

Children and adolescents with disabilities are more likely to be inactive than those without disabilities. Youth with disabilities should work with their healthcare provider to understand the types and amounts of physical activity appropriate for them. When possible, children and adolescents with disabilities should meet the Guidelines. When young people are not able to participate in appropriate physical activities to meet the Guidelines, they should be as active as possible and avoid being inactive.

Chapter 56
Fitness Safety For Girls

Physical Activity Safety Tips

Being active can be great for you and great fun—but not if you get hurt. Stay smart, safe, and strong with our info. On this page, you can find some general physical activity safety tips and learn about warming up and cooling down.

Then keep reading to learn about avoiding injuries like knee problems, concussions, and more. And check out key kinds of safety equipment.

Take These Basic Steps To Stay Safe

- **Be active regularly.** Being active regularly builds fitness, and fit folks have a lower chance of getting hurt.

- **Build up slowly.** Pick activities you can do now, and then slowly challenge yourself. You might add to how often you're active or to how long you're active each time. For example, maybe add five minutes to your workout every week or two.

- **Value variety.** Try to do a mix of activities, so you don't put too much strain on the same parts of your body all the time.

- **Be careful on hot or humid days.** If possible, move your exercise indoors. That's also a good idea on days with a lot of air pollution. If you're going to be outside, rest in the shade, take breaks, and drink lots of water.

About This Chapter: This chapter includes text excerpted from "Physical Activity Safety Tips For Girls," GirlsHealth. gov, Office on Women's Health (OWH), March 27, 2015.

- **Drink plenty of fluids.** You need to drink before, during, and after activity. Read more about what to drink when working out.

- **Find safe places.** Try to stay away from traffic and dark areas, for example. And avoid places with a lot of holes or other things that could make you fall.

- **Follow the rules of the game.** Remember that many of the rules were made just to keep you safe. Learn more about safety in sports.

- **Always use the right safety equipment.** Make sure that your any safety gear fits right and is in good shape.

Warming Up And Cooling Down

Warming up is a good idea. Becoming active too fast can put too much stress on your body. To get going safely, you can just do your activity at a slower pace for 10 minutes.

After you warm up, try stretching your muscles. You also can stretch at the end of your workout. Stretching combined with warming up and strengthening exercises may help prevent injuries. Check out our stretches.

What about a cool-down after being active? Cooling down may not be essential for everyone. Still, stopping suddenly may be risky for some people, and cooling down is pretty simple. If your heart rate and breathing got faster during your workout, your cool-down should slowly get them back to normal. You can do the same activity you were doing, but do it more slowly. For example, if you've been walking fast for 45 minutes, you can walk slowly instead for around 10 minutes.

Avoiding Injuries

Protecting Your Bones

Your teenage years are the most important time for building strong bones. Physical activity, calcium, and vitamin D help build strong bones. Having strong bones can help prevent osteoporosis , which is a disease that can put you at risk for broken bones when you get older.

Sometimes, girls can develop osteoporosis when they're young. This doesn't happen very often. But it can happen if you get a lot of exercise from activities like competitive sports but you don't eat enough healthy food. Osteoporosis can ruin a female athlete's career because it may lead to frequent or serious injuries.

If you exercise a lot like in a competitive sport, make sure to eat a variety of healthy foods, including ones with calcium and vitamin D to protect your bones.

Concussion

A concussion is a type of brain injury. It can happen when your head gets hit. But it also can happen when another part of your body gets hit in a way that the force goes all the way to your brain. Concussion is a possible risk for girls who play basketball, soccer, lacrosse, and other sports.

To lower the chances of getting a concussion, always make sure to follow any rules of your sport and to use the right equipment.

Girls may have different concussion symptoms than boys. In a recent study, girls were more likely to feel drowsy and sensitive to noise. Those signs can be harder to notice than boys' symptoms, which most often were confusion and not remembering things.

If you get a concussion, you must rest your body and your mind. If you think you might have a concussion, you should stop playing right away. If you have a concussion, make sure to follow all your doctor's instructions for healing, even if you start to feel better. When can you play again? When a doctor or other licensed health professional trained in concussions says you can.

Safety Equipment

From helmets to shoes, the right equipment can help keep you safe when playing sports or being active.

Helmets

Helmets help when there's a risk of falling or getting hit in the head, like in baseball, softball, biking, skiing, horseback riding, skateboarding, and inline skating. Make sure you wear a helmet that is made for the activity you are doing. And make sure you know how it is supposed to fit. In some states, the law says you have to wear a helmet while biking. Bike helmets should come with a special sticker from the U.S. Consumer Product Safety Commission (CPSC).

Special Eye Protection

Special eye protection helps prevent many sports-related eye injuries. Sports that have a high risk of eye injury include basketball, baseball, hockey, and racquet sports. Regular glasses or sunglasses will not keep your eyes safe from injury. If you wear regular glasses, the protective eyewear goes over them. If you wear goggles, they should fit snugly and have cushioning for a comfortable fit. Goggles made from a special material called polycarbonate are extremely strong. Ask your coach or eye doctor what type of eye protection you may need.

Mouth Guards

Mouth guards protect your mouth, teeth, and tongue. They offer protection in soccer, lacrosse, basketball, baseball, cheerleading, and other activities in which you could get hit in the mouth. You can get mouth guards at sport stores or from your dentist.

Pads For Your Wrists, Knees, And Elbows

Pads for your wrists, knees, and elbows can help prevent lots of injuries, including broken bones. They are important for activities such as inline skating, snowboarding, and hockey. In some sports, like soccer, your coach may require shin guards, which are pads to protect your lower leg.

Shoes

Shoes need to fit well and be right for your sport. Check with your coach or an athletic shoe salesperson about what shoes to wear. Also ask how often they need to be replaced.

Signs Of Not Eating Enough And Eating Disorders

Sometimes, exercising just lowers a person's appetite. And sometimes limiting food can be a sign that a girl may be developing an eating disorder. Here are some signs that you or a friend may have a problem:

- Worrying about gaining weight if you don't exercise enough
- Trying harder to find time to exercise than to eat
- Chewing gum or drinking water to cope with hunger
- Often wanting to exercise rather than be with friends
- Exercising instead of doing homework or other responsibilities
- Getting very upset if you miss a workout, but not if you miss a meal
- Having people tell you they are worried you are losing too much weight

If you think you or a friend has a problem, talk to a parent, guardian, or trusted adult.

Chapter 57
Mental Fitness

Nutrition And Mental Health

The food you eat can have a direct effect on your energy level, physical health, and mood. A "healthy diet" is one that has enough of each essential nutrient, contains many foods from all of the basic food groups, provides the right amount of calories to maintain a healthy weight, and does not have too much fat, sugar, salt, or alcohol.

By choosing foods that can give you steady energy, you can help your body stay healthy. This may also help your mind feel good. The same diet doesn't work for every person. In order to find the best foods that are right for you, talk to your healthcare professional.

Some vitamins and minerals may help with the symptoms of depression. Experts are looking into how a lack of some nutrients—including folate, vitamin B12, calcium, iron, selenium, zinc, and omega-3—may contribute to depression in new mothers. Ask your doctor or another healthcare professional for more information.

Exercise And Mental Health

Regular physical activity is important to the physical and mental health of almost everyone, including older adults. Being physically active can help you continue to do the things you enjoy and stay independent as you age. Regular physical activity over long periods of time can produce long-term health benefits. That's why health experts say that everyone should be active every day to maintain their health.

About This Chapter: This chapter includes text excerpted from "Good Mental Health," Office on Women's Health (OWH), U.S. Department of Health and Human Services (HHS), March 29, 2010. Reviewed March 2017.

If you are diagnosed with depression or anxiety, your doctor may tell you to exercise in addition to taking any medications or receiving counseling. This is because exercise has been shown to help with the symptoms of depression and anxiety. Your body makes certain chemicals, called endorphins, before and after you work out. They relieve stress and improve your mood. Exercise can also slow or stop weight gain, which is a common side effect of some medications used to treat mental health disorders.

Sleep And Mental Health

Your mind and body will feel better if you sleep well. Your body needs time every day to rest and heal. If you often have trouble sleeping—either falling asleep, or waking during the night and being unable to get back to sleep—one or several of the following ideas might be helpful to you:

- Go to bed at the same time every night and get up at the same time every morning. Avoid "sleeping in" (sleeping much later than your usual time for getting up). It will make you feel worse.

- Establish a bedtime "ritual" by doing the same things every night for an hour or two before bedtime so your body knows when it is time to go to sleep.

- Avoid caffeine, nicotine, and alcohol.

- Eat on a regular schedule and avoid a heavy meal prior to going to bed. Don't skip any meals.

- Eat plenty of dairy foods and dark green leafy vegetables.

- Exercise daily, but avoid strenuous or invigorating activity before going to bed.

- Play soothing music on a tape or compact disc (CD) that shuts off automatically after you are in bed.

- Try a turkey sandwich and a glass of milk before bedtime to make you feel drowsy.

- Try having a small snack before you go to bed, something like a piece of fruit and a piece of cheese, so you don't wake up hungry in the middle of the night. Have a similar small snack if you awaken in the middle of the night.

- Take a warm bath or shower before going to bed.

- Place a drop of lavender oil on your pillow.

- Drink a cup of herbal chamomile tea before going to bed.

You need to see your doctor if:

- You often have difficulty sleeping and the solutions listed above are not working for you

- You awaken during the night gasping for breath

- Your partner says that your breathing stops when you are sleeping

- You snore loudly

- You wake up feeling like you haven't been asleep

- You fall asleep often during the day

Stress And Mental Health

Stress can happen for many reasons. Stress can be brought about by a traumatic accident, death, or emergency situation. Stress can also be a side effect of a serious illness or disease.

There is also stress associated with daily life, the workplace, and family responsibilities. It's hard to stay calm and relaxed in our hectic lives. As women, we have many roles: spouse, mother, caregiver, friend, and/or worker. With all we have going on in our lives, it seems almost impossible to find ways to de-stress. But it's important to find those ways. Your health depends on it.

Common symptoms include:

- Headache

- Sleep disorders

- Difficulty concentrating

- Short-temper

- Upset stomach

- Job dissatisfaction

- Low morale

- Depression

- Anxiety

Remember to always make time for **you**. It's important to care for yourself. Think of this as an order from your doctor, so you don't feel guilty! No matter how busy you are, you can try to set aside at least 15 minutes each day in your schedule to do something for yourself, like taking a bubble bath, going for a walk, or calling a friend.

Chapter 58

Eating Disorders Relapse And Relapse Prevention

What Is A Relapse?

Weight regain usually starts with a **lapse**. A lapse is a brief and small slip in your weight loss efforts.

A lapse might be overeating during dinner for a day or two or skipping your physical activity for a week while you are on vacation. Lapses are a natural part of weight management. At some point, everyone has lapses—small slips, moments, or brief periods of time when they return to an old habit.

REMEMBER that by itself, a lapse will not cause you to gain back the weight you have lost. A relapse is a return to previous eating and activity habits and is associated with significant weight regain.

A lapse left unchecked, however, can grow into a **relapse**. A relapse usually results from a series of several small **lapses** that snowball into a full-blown relapse. The most effective way to prevent a relapse is to identify the lapses early and deal with them before they turn into a relapse.

The Relapse Chain

The **relapse chain** is a series—or chain reaction—of events that can lead to a full relapse. The chain is shown here using the case of "Rose," who slowly but steadily lost 19 pounds during the lifestyle intervention over a seven-month period.

About This Chapter: This chapter includes text excerpted from "Lifestyle Coach Facilitation Guide: Post-Core," Centers for Disease Control and Prevention (CDC), June 14, 2012. Reviewed March 2017.

Rose had adopted healthy eating habits and had made walking a regular part of her week, then the following took place:

- **High risk situation:**

  Rose and her husband went for a long weekend at the beach.

- **No plan for the situation**

  Rose did not plan for how she would maintain her healthy eating and physical activity habits while on vacation.

- **Small lapse occurs**

  Rose decided "on the fly" that she deserved a few days without worrying about what she ate. However, when she got home she weighed herself and couldn't believe that she was two pounds heavier than when she left for her trip!

- **Negative thinking and no plan for lapse**

  Rose became upset at the two pound weight gain and began feeling that there was no use trying anymore. She thought, "If I can't just enjoy myself for a few days, why even bother?"

- **Another relapse and no comeback plan**

  Rose became further depressed and frustrated, and did not resume her healthy eating habits or walking routine.

- **Full relapse**

  A week later, Rose had gained a total of five pounds and decided against going to the scheduled postcore session.

Dealing With Lapses

Step 1: The first step in dealing with lapses is to recognize that 99.9 percent of all **people trying to lose weight and be active experience lapses.** Lapses can and should be useful learning experiences.

Step 2: The second step is to **resist the tendency to think negative thoughts.** You are not a failure if you lapse—you are normal!

Step 3: Next, **ask yourself what happened.** Use the chance to learn from the lapse. *Was it a special occasion? If so, is it likely to happen again soon? Did you eat because of social pressure? Did* *you skip physical activity because you were too busy with other things, or because of work and family pressures?* Review the situation and think about it neutrally. Then plan a strategy for dealing more effectively with similar situations in the future.

Step 4: The fourth step is to **regain control** of your eating or physical activity at the very next opportunity. Do not tell yourself, "Well, I blew it for the day," and wait until the next day to get back on track. Getting back on track without delay is important in preventing lapses from becoming relapses.

Step 5: Talk to someone supportive. Call your Lifestyle Coach, another participant, or another friend or loved one and discuss your new strategy for handling lapses.

Step 6: Finally, **remember you are making lifelong changes.** Weight loss is a journey with lots of small decisions and choices every day that add up over time. Focus on all the positive changes you have made and realize that you can get back on track.

Keeping A Lapse From Becoming A Relapse

In order to deal most effectively with lapses, it is important to be prepared for them.

Present: A lapse (or a single occasion of uncontrolled eating or not being physically active) is not likely—by itself—to cause you to slip back into old habits and regain weight. However, when people eat something they know they shouldn't or stop being active, they often have self-defeating thoughts.

Recognizing High-Risk Situations

Present: Having completed the National Diabetes Prevention Program core sessions, you have probably already been faced with situations where you had to cope with (or think about) lapses. Now that you are in the postcore phase, with a focus on either maintaining your weight or losing additional weight, the high-risk situations you currently face may not be the same as those you faced during the earlier phase of the program.

In addition, situations may not be high-risk across the board. A situation that makes you want to eat high-calorie foods may not affect your physical activity routine and vice versa. Also consider what situations seem to decrease your self-monitoring behavior, which is an easy way to start slipping on eating and activity. Finally, remember that both positive and negative situations can be risky for lapses.

Think about times in the past several weeks when you might have slipped or had a lapse. What was going on? What circumstances led to your lapse?

Planning For Your High-Risk Situations

Part of successful weight management is having a plan to deal with your high-risk situations so that they do not become lapses. **Develop a plan. Write it down.** Look at it when you find yourself faced with a high-risk situation, or in the middle of a slip.

Your plan should involve taking action to change the situation, your thoughts and behaviors, or both. Make sure your plan is specific and detailed, so that you will be able to follow it when you are in the middle of a high-risk situation.

Planning For Comeback

Keep these things in mind while planning your comeback:

- Reflect on your progress. Remember your purpose.

- Remember that a short period of overeating or skipped activity will not erase all of your progress.

- Be kind to yourself. Stay calm and listen to your positive self-talk (while sending negative thoughts away). How you think about your lapse is the most important part of the process. If you use it as a learning opportunity, you will succeed. If you give up and stop trying to make changes, then you are at risk for a relapse.

Think about what will be the most effective comeback plan for you to recover from a lapse and prevent a full relapse. Write down these steps and keep your written plan in a place where you can easily find it when you need it.

Part Six
If You Need More Information

Chapter 59

For More Information About Eating Disorders

Academy for Eating Disorders (AED)

11130 Sunrise Valley Dr.
Ste. 350
Reston, VA 20191
Phone: 703-234-4079
Fax: 703-435-4390
Website: www.aedweb.org
E-mail: info@aedweb.org

The Alliance for Eating Disorders Awareness

1649 Forum Pl.
Ste. 2
West Palm Beach, FL 33401
Toll-Free: 866-662-1235
Phone: 561-841-0900
Fax: 561-653-0043
Website: www.allianceforeatingdisorders.com/portal/contact-us
E-mail: info@allianceforeatingdisorders.com

Binge Eating Disorder Association (BEDA)

637 Emerson Pl.
Severna Park, MD 21146
Phone: 855-855-BEDA (855-855-2332)
Fax: 410-741-3037
Website: www.bedaonline.com

About This Chapter: Resources in this chapter were compiled from several sources deemed reliable; all contact information was verified and updated in March 2017.

Bulimia Nervosa Resource Guide

ECRI Institute
5200 Butler Pike
Plymouth Meeting, PA 19462
Website: www.bulimiaguide.org
E-mail: htais@ecri.org

Caring Online

Toll-Free: 888-884-4913
Phone: 425-771-5166
Website: www.caringonline.com

Casa Palmera Treatment Center

14750 El Camino Real
Del Mar, CA 92014
Toll-Free: 888-481-4481
Website: www.casapalmera.com

Children's Hospital Colorado

Anschutz Medical Campus
13123 E. 16th Ave.
Aurora, CO 80045
Toll-Free: 800-624-6553
Phone: 720-777-0123
Website: www.childrenscolorado.org

Eating Disorder Hope (EDH)™

8520 Golden Pheasant Ct.
Redmond, OR 97756
Website: www.eatingdisorderhope.com
E-mail: info@eatingdisorderhope.com

The Eating Disorder Foundation

1901 E. 20th Ave.
Denver, CO 80205
Phone: 303-322-3373
Fax: 303-322-3364
Website: www.eatingdisorderfoundation.org
E-mail: info@eatingdisorderfoundation.org

Eating Disorders Coalition (EDC)
P.O. Box 96503-98807
Washington, DC 20090
Phone: 202-543-9570
Website: www.eatingdisorderscoalition.org
E-mail: manager@eatingdisorderscoalition.org

Eating Disorders Foundation of Victoria (EDV)
Collingwood Football Club Community Centre
cnr Lulie and Abbot Streets
Abbotsford VIC 3067
Australia
Phone:(1300 550 236; (03) 9417 6598)
Fax: 394-175-787
Website: www.eatingdisorders.org.au
E-mail: help@eatingdisorders.org.au

Eating Recovery Center (ERC)
7351 E. Lowry Blvd.
Ste. 200
Denver, CO 80230
Toll-Free: 877-711-1690
Website: www.eatingrecoverycenter.com
E-mail: info@eatingrecoverycenter.com

EDReferral.com
Website: www.edreferral.com

F.E.A.S.T. (Families Empowered and Supporting Treatment of Eating Disorders)
P.O. Box 1281
Warrenton, VA 20185
Toll-Free: 855-50-FEAST (855-503-3278)
Website: www.feast-ed.org
E-mail: info@feast-ed.org

Female Athlete Triad Coalition
Website: www.femaleathletetriad.org

The Harris Center for Education and Advocacy in Eating Disorders

2 Longfellow Pl.
Ste. 200
Boston, MA 02114
Phone: 617-726-8470
Fax: 617-726-1595

Mirror-Mirror

Website: www.mirror-mirror.org

Multi-Service Eating Disorders Association (MEDA)

288 Walnut St.
Ste. 130
Newton, MA 02460
Phone: 617-558-1881
Website: www.medainc.org

National Association of Anorexia Nervosa and Associated Disorders (ANAD)

750 E. Diehl Rd.
Ste. 127
Naperville, IL 60563
Phone: 630-577-1333
Website: www.anad.org
E-mail: hello@anad.org

National Center for Overcoming Overeating

Website: www.overcomingovereating.com

National Eating Disorder Information Centre (NEDIC)

ES 7-421, 200 Elizabeth St.
Toronto, ON M5G 2C4
Canada
Toll-Free: 866-NEDIC-20 (866-633-4220)
Phone: 416-340-4156
Fax: 416-340-4736
Website: www.nedic.ca
E-mail: nedic@uhn.ca

National Eating Disorders Association (NEDA)
165 W. 46th St.
Ste. 402
New York, NY 10036
Toll-Free: 800-931-2237
Phone: 212-575-6200
Fax: 212-575-1650
Website: www.nationaleatingdisorders.org
E-mail: info@NationalEatingDisorders.org

Overeaters Anonymous
6075 Zenith Ct. N.E.
Rio Rancho, NM 87144-6424
Phone: 505-891-2664
Fax: 505-891-4320
Website: www.oa.org

Rader Programs
Toll-Free: 800-841-1515
Website: www.raderprograms.com

Remuda Ranch
1245 Jack Burden Rd.
Wickenburg, AZ 85390
Toll-Free: 800-445-1900
Phone: 866-332-2919
Website: www.remudaranch.com

River Centre Clinic
5465 Main St.
Sylvania, OH 43560
Toll-Free: 877-212-5457
Phone: 419-885-8800
Fax: 419-885-8600
Website: www.river-centre.org
E-mail: info@river-centre.org

Sheena's Place

87 Spadina Rd.
Toronto, ON M5R 2T1
Canada
Phone: 416-927-8900
Fax: 416-927-8844
Website: www.sheenasPl..org
E-mail: info@sheenasPl..org

Something Fishy

Website: www.something-fishy.org

Chapter 60

For More Information About Nutrition And Weight Management

Academy of Nutrition and Dietetics

120 South Riverside Plaza
Ste. 2190
Chicago, IL 60606-6995
Toll-Free: 800-877-1600
Phone: 312-899-0040
Website: www.eatrightpro.org

American Diabetes Association

2451 Crystal Dr.
Ste. 900
Arlington, VA 22202
Toll-Free: 800-DIABETES (800-342-2383)
Website: www.diabetes.org
E-mail: askada@diabetes.org

American Heart Association

7272 Greenville Ave.
Dallas, TX 75231
Toll-Free: 800-AHA-USA1 (800-242-8721)
Website: www.heart.org

Ask the Dietitian®

Website: www.dietitian.com

About This Chapter: Resources in this chapter were compiled from several sources deemed reliable; all contact information was verified and updated in March 2017.

Center for Science in the Public Interest (CSPI)

1220 L St. N.W.
Ste. 300
Washington, DC 20005
Phone: 202-332-9110
Fax: 202-265-4954
Website: www.cspinet.org
E-mail: cspi@cspinet.org

Centers for Disease Control and Prevention (CDC)

Division of Nutrition, Physical Activity, and Obesity (DNPAO)
1600 Clifton Rd.
Atlanta, GA 30329-4027
Toll-Free: 800-CDC-INFO (800-232-4636)
TTY: 888-232-6348
Website: www.cdc.gov/nccdphp/dnpao/

ChooseMyPlate.gov

USDA Center for Nutrition Policy and Promotion
3101 Park Center Dr.
Alexandria, VA 22302-1594
Website: www.choosemyplate.gov

Eunice Kennedy Shriver National Institute of Child Health and Human Development (NICHD)

P.O. Box 3006
Rockville, MD 20847
Toll-Free: 800-370-2943
Toll-Free TTY: 888-320-6942
Fax: 866-760-5947
Website: www.nichd.nih.gov
E-mail: NICHDInformationResourceCenter@mail.nih.gov

Food and Nutrition Information Center (FNIC)

National Agricultural Library
10301 Baltimore Ave.
Beltsville, MD 20705
Phone: 301-504-5755
Website: www.fnic.nal.usda.gov
E-mail: fnic@ars.usda.gov

GirlsHealth.gov
Office on Women's Health (OWH) U.S. Department of Health and Human Services (HHS)
200 Independence Ave. S.W.
Rm. 712E
Washington, DC 20201
Website: www.girlshealth.gov

International Food Information Council (IFIC) Foundation
1100 Connecticut Ave. N.W.
Ste. 430
Washington, DC 20036
Phone: 202-296-6540
Website: www.foodinsight.org
E-mail: info@foodinsight.org

KidsHealth®
The Nemours Foundation
10140 Centurion Pkwy
Jacksonville, FL 32256
Phone: 904-697-4100
Website: www.kidshealth.org

National Agricultural Library (NAL)
Food and Nutrition Information Center
10301 Baltimore Ave.
Beltsville, MD 20705
Website: www.nal.usda.gov

National Center for Complementary and Integrative Health (NCCIH)
NCCIH Clearinghouse
P.O. Box 7923
Gaithersburg, MD 20898-7923
Toll-Free: 888-644-6226
Toll-Free TTY: 866-464-3615
Fax: 866-464-3616
Website: www.nccih.nih.gov

National Heart, Lung, and Blood Institute (NHLBI)

NHLBI Health Information Center
P.O. Box 30105
Bethesda, MD 20824-0105
Phone: 301-592-8573
TTY: 240-629-3255
Fax: 301-592-8563
Website: www.nhlbi.nih.gov
E-mail: nhlbiinfo@ nhlbi.nih.gov

National Women's Health Information Center (NWHIC)

Office on Women's Health (OWH), U.S. Department of Health and Human Services
(HHS)
200 Independence Ave. S.W.
Washington, DC 20201
Toll-free: 800-994-9662
Phone: 202-690-7650
Toll-Free TDD: 888-220-5446
Fax: 202-205-2631
Website: www.womenshealth.gov

The Obesity Society

1110 Bonifant St.
Ste. 500
Silver Spring, MD 20910
Phone: 301-563-6526
Fax: 301-563-6595
Website: www.obesity.org

Office of Dietary Supplements (ODS)

National Institutes of Health
6100 Executive Blvd.
Rm. 3B01, MSC 7517
Bethesda, MD 20892-7517
Phone: 301-435-2920
Fax: 301-480-1845
Website: www.ods.od.nih.gov
E-mail: ods@nih.gov

U.S. Department of Agriculture (USDA)

1400 Independence Ave. S.W.
Washington, DC 20250
Phone: 202-720-2791
TDD: 202-720-2600
Website: www.usda.gov
E-mail: agsec@usda.gov

U.S. Food and Drug Administration (FDA)

10903 New Hampshire Ave.
Silver Spring, MD 20993
Toll-Free: 888-INFO-FDA (888-463-6332)
Phone: 301-796-4540
Fax: 301-847-8622
Website: www.fda.gov

Vegetarian Resource Group (VRG)

P.O. Box 1463
Baltimore, MD 21203
Phone: 410-366-8343
Website: www.vrg.org
E-mail: vrg@vrg.org

Weight-Control Information Network (WIN)

National Institute of Diabetes and Digestive and Kidney Diseases
1 WIN Way
Bethesda, MD 20892-3665
Toll-Free: 877-946-4627
Fax: 202-828-1028
Website: www.niddk.nih.gov/health-information/health-communication-programs/win/
Pages/default.aspx
E-mail: win@info.niddk.nih.gov

Chapter 61

For More Information About Physical And Mental Fitness

Physical Fitness And Exercise

Action for Healthy Kids

600 W. Van Buren St.
Ste. 720
Chicago, IL 60607
Toll-Free: 800-416-5136
Fax: 312-212-0098
Website: www.actionforhealthykids.org

Aerobics and Fitness Association of America (AFAA)

1750 E. Northrop Blvd.
Ste. 200
Chandler, AZ 85286
Toll-Free: 800-446-2322
Website: www.afaa.com

The American Council on Exercise (ACE)

4851 Paramount Dr.
San Diego, CA 92123
Toll-Free: 888-825-3636
Phone: 858-576-6500
Fax: 858-576-6564
Website: www.acefitness.org
E-mail: support@acefitness.org

About This Chapter: Resources in this chapter were compiled from several sources deemed reliable; all contact information was verified and updated in March 2017.

American Health and Fitness Alliance

P.O. Box 7827
Pine Island WPB, FL 33411
Phone: 212-808-0765
Fax: 212-988-3130
Website: www.health-fitness.org
E-mail: order@health-fitness.org

American Running Association (ARA)

4405 East-West Hwy
Ste. 405
Bethesda, MD 20814
Phone: 800-776-2732 (ext. 13 or ext. 12)
Fax: 301-913-9520
Website: www.americanrunning.org

Aquatic Exercise Association (AEA)

201 Tamiami Trail S.
Ste. 3
Nokomis, FL 34275
Toll-Free: 888-232-9283
Phone: 941-486-8600
Website: www.aeawave.com

Centers for Disease Control and Prevention (CDC)

Division of Nutrition, Physical Activity, and Obesity (DNPAO)
1600 Clifton Rd.
Atlanta, GA 30329-4027
Toll-Free: 800-CDC-INFO (800-232-4636)
Toll-Free TTY: 888-232-6348
Website: www.cdc.gov/nccdphp/dnpao/index.html

Fitness Institute Australia (FIA)

Level 3, 815-825 George St.
Sydney NSW 2000
Australia
Toll-Free: 300-136-632
Phone: 282-047-800
Fax: 292-804-948
Website: www.fiafitnation.com.au
E-mail: info@fiafitnation.com.au

Girls Health

U.S. Department of Health and Human Services
200 Independence Ave. S.W.
Rm. 712E
Washington, DC 20201
Website: www.girlshealth.gov

HealthyWomen

P.O. Box 430
Red Bank, NJ 07701
Toll-Free: 877-986-9472
Phone: 732-530-3425
Fax: 732-865-7225
Website: www.healthywomen.org
E-mail: info@healthywomen.org

IDEA Health & Fitness Association

10190 Telesis Ct.
San Diego, CA 92121
Toll-Free: 800-999-4332 (ext. 7)
Phone: 858-535-8979 (ext. 7)
Fax: 619-344-0380
Website: www.ideafit.com
E-mail: contact@ideafit.com

International Fitness Association (IFA)

12472 Lake Underhill Rd.
Ste. 341
Orlando, FL 32828-7144
Toll-Free: 800-227-1976
Phone: 407-579-8610
Website: www.ifafitness.com

International Health, Racquet and Sportsclub Association (IHRSA)

70 Fargo St.
Boston, MA 02210
Toll-Free: 800-228-4772
Phone: 617-951-0055
Fax: 617-951-0056
Website: www.ihrsa.org
E-mail: info@ihrsa.org

KidsHealth®

The Nemours Foundation
10140 Centurion Pkwy
Jacksonville, FL 32256
Phone: 904-697-4100
Fax: 904-697-4220
Website: www.nemours.org

LiveStrong

2201 E. Sixth St.
Austin, TX 78702
Toll-Free: 877-236-8820
Phone: 855-220-7777
Website: www.livestrong.org

National Alliance for Youth Sports (NAYS)

2050 Vista Pkwy
West Palm Beach, FL 33411
Toll-Free: 800-729-2057
Phone: 800-688-5437
Fax: 561-684-2546
Website: www.nays.org
E-mail: nays@nays.org

National Coalition for Promoting Physical Activity (NCPPA)

1150 Connecticut Ave. N.W.
Ste. 300
Washington, DC 20036
Website: www.ncppa.org
E-mail: ayanna@ncppa.org

National Institute for Fitness and Sport (NIFS)

250 University Blvd.
Indianapolis, IN 46202
Phone: 317-274-3432
Fax: 317-274-7408
Website: www.nifs.org

National Recreation and Park Association (NRPA)

22377 Belmont Ridge Rd.
Ashburn, VA 20148-4501
Toll-Free: 800-626-NRPA (800-626-6772)
Website: www.nrpa.org

National Strength and Conditioning Association (NSCA)

1885 Bob Johnson Dr.
Colorado Springs, CO 80906
Toll-Free: 800-815-6826
Phone: 719-632-6722
Fax: 719-632-6367
Website: www.nsca.com
E-mail: nsca@nsca-lift.org

PE Central

2516 Blossom Trl W.
Blacksburg, VA 24060
Phone: 540-953-1043
Fax: 866-776-9170
Website: www.pecentral.org

President's Council on Fitness, Sports and Nutrition (PCFSN)

1101 Wootton Pkwy
Ste. 560
Rockville, MD 20852
Phone: 240-276-9567
Fax: 240-276-9860
Website: www.fitness.gov
E-mail: fitness@hhs.gov

SHAPE (Society of Health and Physical Educators) America

1900 Association Dr.
Reston, VA 20191
Phone: 800-213-7193
Fax: 703-476-9527
Website: www.aahperd.org

Spark Teens

Website: www.sparkteens.com

SportsMD

Phone: 203-689-6880
Website: www.sportsmd.com
E-mail: contactus@sportsmd.com

Women's Sports Foundation

247 W. 30th St.
Ste. 7R
New York, NY 10001
Toll-Free: 800-227-3988
Phone: 646-845-0273
Fax: 212-967-757
Website: www.womenssportsfoundation.org
E-mail: Info@WomensSportsFoundation.org

Mental Wellness

American Academy of Child and Adolescent Psychiatry (AACAP)

3615 Wisconsin Ave. N.W.
Washington, DC 20016-3007
Phone: 202-966-7300
Fax: 202-464-0131
Website: www.aacap.org

American Counseling Association (ACA)

6101 Stevenson Ave.
Alexandria, VA 22304
Toll-Free: 800-347-6647
Toll-Free Fax: 800-473-2329
Fax: 703-823-0252
Website: www.counseling.org
E-mail: webmaster@counseling.org.

American Psychiatric Association

1000 Wilson Blvd.
Ste. 1825
Arlington, VA 22209-3901
Toll-Free: 888-35-PSYCH (888-357-7924)
Phone: 703-907-7300
Website: www.psych.org
E-mail: apa@psych.org

American Psychological Association (APA)

750 First St. N.E.
Washington, DC 20002-4242
Toll-Free: 800-374-2721
Phone: 202-336-5500
TDD: 202-336-6123
Website: www.apa.org

Association for Behavioral and Cognitive Therapies (ABCT)

305 7th Ave. 16th Fl.
New York, NY 10001
Phone: 212-647-1890
Fax: 212-647-1865
Website: www.abct.org

Canadian Mental Health Association

500-250 Dundas St. W.
Toronto, ON M5T 2Z5
Canada
Phone: 613-745-7750
Fax: 613-745-5522
Website: www.cmha.ca
E-mail: Info@cmha.ca

Canadian Psychological Association (CPA)

141 Laurier Ave. W.
Ste. 702
Ottawa, ON K1P 5J3
Toll-Free: 888-472-0657
Phone: 613-237-2144
Fax: 613-237-1674
Website: www.cpa.ca

Center for Mental Health Services (CMHS)

Substance Abuse and Mental Health Services Administration
5600 Fishers Ln.
Rockville, MD 20857
Toll-Free: 877-SAMHSA-7 (877-726-4727)
Phone: 240-276-1310
Fax: 301-480-8491
Website: www.samhsa.gov

Centre for Clinical Interventions

223 James St.
Northbridge, Western Australia 6003
Australia
Phone: 089-227-4399
Fax: 089-328-5911
Website: www.cci.health.wa.gov.au
E-mail: info.cci@health.wa.gov.au

Mental Health America (MHA)

(formerly National Mental Health Assn.)
500 Montgomery St.
Ste. 820
Alexandria, VA 22314
Toll-Free: 800-969-6642
Phone: 703-684-7722
Fax: 703-684-5968
Website: www.nmha.org

Mind

15-19 Bdwy.
Stratford, London E15 4BQ
Phone: 208-519-2122
Fax: 208-522-1725
Website: www.mind.org.uk
E-mail: supporterservices@mind.org.uk

National Alliance on Mental Illness (NAMI)

3803 N. Fairfax Dr.
Ste. 100
Arlington, VA 22203
Toll-Free: 800-950-6264
Phone: 703-524-7600
Website: www.nami.org
E-mail: info@nami.org

National Institute of Mental Health (NIMH)

6001 Executive Blvd.
Rm. 6200, MSC 9663
Bethesda, MD 20892-9663
Toll-Free: 866-615-6464
Phone: 301-443-4513
TTY: 301-443-8431
Fax: 301-443-4279
Website: www.nimh.nih.gov
E-mail: nimhinfo@nih.gov

Psych Central

55 Pleasant St.
Ste. 207
Newburyport, MA 01950
Website: www.psychcentral.com

Royal College of Psychiatrists

21 Prescot St.
London E1 8BB
Phone: 207-235-2351
Fax: 0203-701-2761
Website: www.rcpsych.ac.uk
E-mail: reception@rcpsych.ac.uk

Substance Abuse and Mental Health Services Administration (SAMHSA)

5600 Fishers Ln.
Rockville, MD 20857
Toll-Free: 877-SAMHSA-7 (877-726-4727)
Toll-Free TDD: 800-487-4889
Website: www.samhsa.gov

Index

Index

Page numbers that appear in *Italics* refer to tables or illustrations. Page numbers that have a small 'n' after the page number refer to citation information shown as Notes. Page numbers that appear in **Bold** refer to information contained in boxes within the chapters.